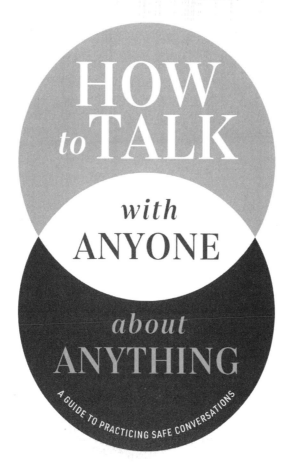

HOW to TALK

with ANYONE

about ANYTHING

A GUIDE TO PRACTICING SAFE CONVERSATIONS

WORKBOOK

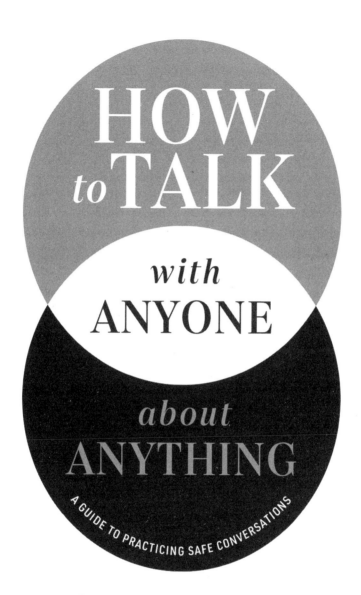

HOW to TALK

with ANYONE

about ANYTHING

A GUIDE TO PRACTICING SAFE CONVERSATIONS

WORKBOOK

HARVILLE HENDRIX, Ph.D. & HELEN LaKELLY HUNT, Ph.D.

New York Times Bestselling Authors

W Publishing Group

An Imprint of Thomas Nelson

Printed in the United States of America
24 25 26 27 28 LBC 5 4 3 2 1

Contents

Introduction

How to Talk with Anyone about Anything introduced you to the concept of "relational competency" (RC), which we defined as "the ability to interact successfully with others by engaging and connecting beyond our differences." Sounds relatively simple, right? And something we should strive for (or we may already feel we are quite competent enough). It's the "beyond our differences" part of the definition that often becomes problematic. It's easier to interact with others who are like-minded—same moral values, faith, nationality, gender, race, eating habits, political affiliation, marital status, and so on.

Our world is made up of groups formed because they found common ground. Parents of adults with high-functioning autism. Low-carb support groups. *SpongeBob SquarePants* meme Facebook groups. The Luxuriant, Flowing Hair Club for Scientists. If you can imagine it, it's there. And even those groups break down into smaller groups with additional delineations. The bubble gets smaller as we look for replicas of ourselves, so they don't challenge who we are.

Differences can be scary. They tap into the unknown, upset the status quo, and threaten our existence. Differences, however, are the defining feature of nature. There is no sameness in the universe, only similarity. Only differences exist. Sameness would, in fact, leave any living thing vulnerable to extinction. Every "thing" is made up of a polarity, two things that are different—like the sperm and egg that produced you. We and everything else arise from interactions between two things that are different. Differences protect us and invite psychological, emotional, biological, and spiritual growth.

As humans, we have a choice: to polarize around difference or to accept difference and use the tension between to generate enormous creativity. We can avoid or shut out disagreement and become isolated, or we can tap into curiosity and embrace empathy. Tension around differences can also inform us about ourselves, because often, tension has a story "in here" rather than "over there."

This workbook will give you skills and strategies to help you move into curiosity and empathy when you disagree with someone. It will also help you unravel the layers under conflict to discover your inner narratives and triggers that contribute to relational tension.

From Me to You to We

Many of our interactions are transactional. We make deals. I win and you lose. This is based on our culture of individualism. We enter any relationship with an egocentric attitude: *What can this person* offer *me? How can they make me* feel better *about myself? How can I get them to see how* great *I really am? How can I convince them of my* rightness? These inner narratives contribute to what we all desire: to be seen, heard, and valued as we truly are—the authentic self. Not being seen, heard, and valued triggers the painful sensation of anxiety, the fear that *I don't exist* or *I am not good enough*; our defenses are activated, and we become polarized. But the overfocus on individualism, while necessary to break from our feudal history, has caused the loneliness, conflict, and polarization that are plaguing our world today.

Here's the catch. To be seen, we must first see. To be heard, we must first hear. To be valued, we must first value. When we encounter another—whether it's at the supermarket, at work, at home—we need to shift our attitudes toward the other: *What can I learn here? What don't I know?* Listening to truly understand those around you, being curious about them, and responding with awe, draws others to you. When another person feels seen, heard, and valued, they feel physically and emotionally safe. Defenses drop. Then they see you as a friend rather than foe.

Putting our thoughts and feelings aside momentarily is not easy. But developing relational competency provides the opportunity to develop healthy relationships. And on this journey toward relational competency, an amazing response occurs. We are joyfully relaxed, fully alive, and, above all, *connected*. We then have a greater capacity to love. It starts with "I," moves to "you," and then becomes "we" as we travel a spiral path with a greater propensity to care for others and for the whole of humanity.

The Four Pillars of Safe Conversations

Relational competency is the capacity to create and maintain consistent and positive connections with another person. It is a pathway that involves four practices:

1. **A structured dialogue:** Learning a new way to talk and listen to one another—individually or in a group setting—despite our differences. This is more like a foundation rather than a pillar. Without this, the house is unsteady and the architect wonders what went wrong. With this, the architect joyfully lives inside, connected to the outside world.

2. **Empathy with everyone:** Practicing and growing our ability to empathize. While we are empathic at birth, our early experiences tend to truncate the ability to feel for another. But we can regain this important capacity through simple practices. Empathy can be learned.

3. **The Zero Negativity commitment:** Avoiding negativity at all times involves eliminating put-downs, name-calling, eye rolls, and any other form of shame, blame, or criticism of anyone with whom you communicate each day.

4. **The practice of affirmations:** Affirmation is the acknowledgment of the intrinsic value of another person, not because they did something for us, but because they "exist." To affirm another person is to accept them unconditionally and to celebrate that person's authentic self. The practice of affirmations helps sustain connecting, full aliveness, relaxed joyfulness, and wonder in all relationships.

Within these pillars are sub-learnings, such as cultivating curiosity, increasing our awareness of our defense patterns, and understanding how conflict is an opportunity for growth. All these practices are universal for everyone everywhere—working, learning, worshiping, and living. Once we practice and master these relational skills, we become a social *being* influencer, which is much better than a social media influencer. Social being influencers seek engagement with others rather than fame and fortune based on capitalistic tendencies. Social being influencers see everyone as fragile yet an awesome piece of the amazing whole. Social being influencers do not leave trails of wounding footprints when walking away from others but create connections when walking toward and with them. These meaningful connections define our purpose.

Getting Started

This workbook is organized into eight sessions to cultivate our ability to master the four pillars. Most sessions include the following in some variety:

- Review: for in-depth learnings, review the material in *How to Talk with Anyone about Anything*
- Introduction: an overview of the section's learnings
- Read: passages to read to deepen your understanding
- Write: written exercises to develop the skills and provide insights
- Dialogue: dialogue practices to hone the skills
- Practice: an exercise to practice the skills discussed
- Me-2-We Journal: prompts for writing in a journal
- Daily Do: daily practices

To become relationally competent, we recommend you spend at least one week on each section before you move on to another practice. But you will be the best judge of whether you need more or less time. Complete each session in the order that it is written and don't skip a week, so you can maintain your momentum and integrate the skills you are practicing.

Session 8 takes these skills and applies them into four areas of your life: working, learning, worshiping, and living (that is, your everyday life).

The Concept of Stretching

Homeostasis is a process built into living things to maintain an inner equilibrium. It's a self-regulating system that offsets any change to keep internal states stable and balanced and is nature's elegant design to keep us alive. Change, therefore, can be a warning sign to our basic instincts. The problem with homeostasis, however, is that it does not distinguish between a good change and a bad one. It's why we recommend repeating behaviors for at least sixty days for a new behavior to become habitual.

This work requires us to change in ways that might be uncomfortable. It requires us to stretch beyond our comfort level and move into new behaviors. While we might meet resistance along the way, with consistent practice, new behaviors will ultimately become a part of our makeup. However, we don't want to stretch to the extent where we will quit. It's the Goldilocks of the relational journey: not too soft (easy) where nothing discernible happens, not too hard (impossible) where you break down and sabotage your relationships, but just right (doable but stretches us a bit). The healthy medium is stretching into new behaviors that are small, achievable, and sustainable that strengthen our relational muscle.

At times, an inner voice might warn you. It might tell you something like, *Stop! This is ridiculous!* or *Why should I do all the work?* or *I'm too tired for this fluff!* That is normal, and if you feel this way along this journey, you might say, "I recognize you. Thank you for the warning." And continue doing what you are doing.

How to Proceed

- **Read all of** *How to Talk with Anyone about Anything* before session 1. This will provide the overview for the work.
- **Purchase a writing journal.** While there are pages in this workbook for your journal writings, we encourage you to purchase a separate journal and label it "Me-2-We Journey." Throughout this workbook there will be prompts for your Me-2-We Journey. Spend a minimum of five minutes a day writing in your journal. You can either choose your own thought to write about or use one of the prompts provided. This is purely for you to freely express your thoughts on paper and help create a relational mindset.
- **Identify a practice partner.** While you can do much of the work on your own, it's better to invite a friend or a relative to walk this journey with you. Your practice partner will need their own workbook and book.
  - ~ Good: doing the workbook on your own. Please note, though, that without a Safe Conversations Dialogue partner, you will not be able to complete all the exercises.
  - ~ Better: doing the workbook with your friend or relative.
  - ~ Best: doing this workbook with your intimate other.
- **Commit to learning.** Spend at least thirty minutes a day reading the passages and completing the written work, and choose what time of the day you will do this. Is it every

morning at seven? Is it every evening after dinner at six thirty? If you can't do it daily, schedule a commitment that works for you and is achievable.

- **Commit to practicing.** Identify with your partner the time and the amount of time you can connect for Dialogue practices. Again, ideally this is thirty minutes a day, but even a short daily exchange is better than none. If you are not working with a partner, you can still commit to thirty minutes on Dialogue practices.

The Tipping Point

While relational competency is the achievement, SC Dialogue is the process that, once integrated into our lives, becomes the next shift in human social evolution. It moves us from monologue, which has dominated our human history, to dialogue, which is arising out of the collective unconscious as the need to save our planet and our species reaches a critical level. We believe our SC methodology and tools are more than a new way to communicate. They are the path to a new way of living together that will enhance the lives of everyone and be an invitation to experiencing connection and belonging. The welfare of each of us is dependent upon the welfare of us all. These skills offer a new way to talk without criticism, to listen without judgment, and to connect beyond our differences.

Small changes have big impacts. If enough people practice this way of being, then we reach a critical mass, a tipping point where there is a cultural shift. We move from individuals *teaching* to a civilization *being*. When we can work and live together despite our differences, we will be on a path to a new relational civilization that values universal freedom, full equality for everyone, the celebration of diversity, and total inclusiveness. We wish you well on this relational journey.

When you are ready to begin, first read and sign the My Commitment to the Relational Competency Journey on the following page.

Harville & Helen

My Commitment to the Relational Competency Journey

I, _____, understand that the quality of my relationships determines the quality of my life. I sign this statement of commitment as an indication of my willingness to participate in this relational journey to become more relationally competent in the relationships that define my life.

I agree to:

- spend a minimum of thirty minutes a day working on new learnings (reading and writing worksheets).
- spend a minimum of ten minutes a day practicing Dialogue skills.
- spend a minimum of five minutes a day writing in my Me-2-We Journal.
- complete the work in the order that it is presented in this workbook.
- actively participate in the entire process to the best of my ability.
- stretch a little throughout this journey into new behaviors and practices but not too much to break me.

Optional: _____ has agreed to be my practice partner on this journey. I agree to support my partner's journey without shame, blame, or criticism, knowing they are also seeking to be relationally competent and doing the best they can.

Signature: _____

Date: _____

Setting the Path to Relational Competency

Review: Introduction, Chapters 1–2

Introduction

Everyone has an implicit relational dream. It is housed in the right brain in the form of images that can be accessed by the language resources of the left brain with questions like, "What do your relationships look like?" and "How do they make you feel?" What the brain can imagine, it can put into words. And what it can put into words, it can use to design actions that create the ideal experience that is portrayed in the imagination. Additionally, whatever you focus on is what you get! If you look at the glass as half-empty, you will feel the pain of what is missing in your life. If you look at the glass as half-full, you will feel grateful for life's abundance.

Session 1 focuses on exploring your narratives about relationships, identifying your relationships, assessing your current relational competency skills, and mapping out your relationship goals. It means asking yourself questions like, *What am I trying to achieve? Do I want to be a better leader at work? Or a better friend? A relationally competent parent who is raising relationally competent children?* With a map in hand, you are less likely to get lost on your journey. Let's begin.

Write: My Relational Inventory

Purpose: To identify your current inner narratives (how you think and feel) about relationships.

Instructions: Read through these sentences and fill in the blanks.

What I learned when reading *How to Talk with Anyone about Anything* is _____ _____.

When I think about Safe Conversations (SC) Dialogue and becoming relationally competent and taking this journey:

I feel _____,

and I think _____,

and my body reacts to this by _____.

My listening skills are _____.

I relate to strangers by _____.

I handle conflict by _____.

What I love most about people is _____.

What I despise most about people is _____.

I think work relationships are _____.

I think family relationships are _____.

I feel gratitude when _____.

I express appreciation with others by _____.

My friends are _____.

A relationship that I particularly want to improve is _____.

A relationship that gives me real joy is _____.

A relationship that challenges me is _____.

When someone expresses an opinion I don't agree with,

I say _____,

I feel _____, and

I react _____.

Me-2-We Journey: Relational Me

Using one of the following prompts or stream of consciousness, spend at least five minutes writing what comes to mind in the space below (or write in your separate Me-2-We Journal).

The part in my relational life that works well is . . .

The part in my relational life that needs improvement is . . .

Write: My Relational Bubbles

Purpose: To help you be mindful of all the relationships around you that you may take for granted, and identify opportunities for practicing your relational competency (RC) skills throughout this journey.

Overview: Our lives are made up of relationships. We cannot *not* be in relationship. Even our cells in our bodies are in relationship. There is no such thing as a separate entity. We commingle, share, and interact. And even if we are not consciously aware, every interaction alters how we think and feel, creating experiential memories that inform how we relate to others.

Instructions:

1. Think about the relationships in your life—people in your immediate and extended family; friends; coworkers and employer; fellow students and teachers at school; people you interact with during your daily routines, such as the security guard in your lobby, the crosswalk guard at your daughter's school, or your neighbors.

2. Using the circles on the next two pages, list people using the following ratings:
   - ~ EASY: Effortless. No or little tension. Enjoyable. Can include people I admire.
   - ~ NEUTRAL: People I don't know much about but I see regularly (for example, people at work, in retail stores you visit regularly, or on your daily walks).
   - ~ CHALLENGING: Closer relationships that are tense.
   - ~ IMPOSSIBLE: People I avoid at all costs. Upsets/angers me just to think about them. Don't want them at my dinner table.
     - » Note: If there are people that fall between two areas, you can write their names in the overlapping circles.

3. In the Easy bubble, circle the top three relationships that give you the most joy.

4. In the Impossible bubble, circle the three relationships that are the most difficult.

EASY

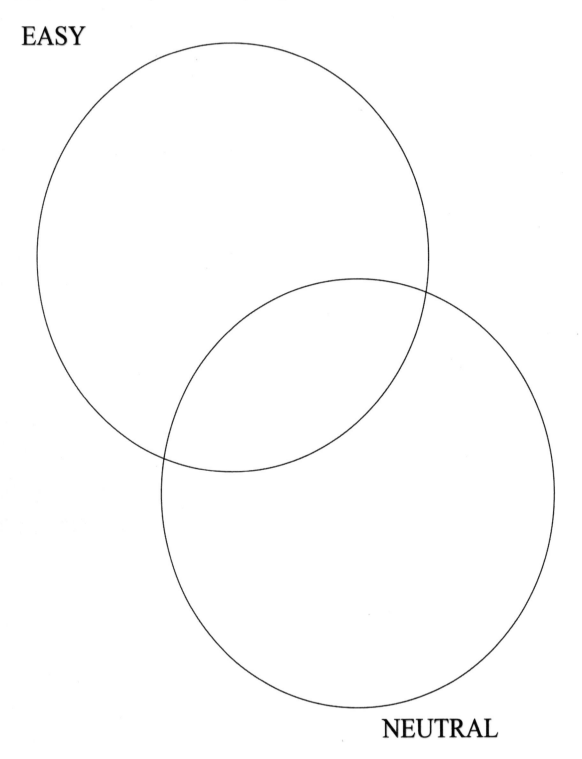

NEUTRAL

CHALLENGING

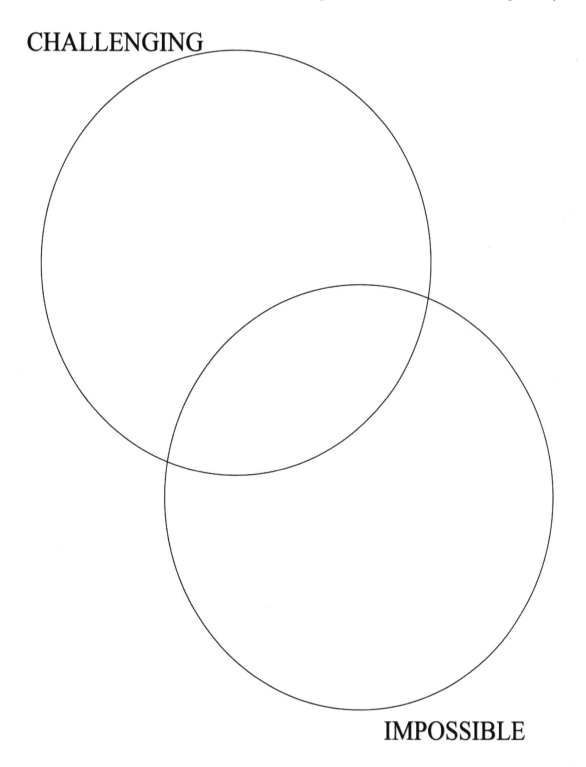

IMPOSSIBLE

Write: My Relational Profile

Instructions:

1. In the following table, list traits you admire in the positive column and traits you dislike in the negative column. Use adjectives such as *kind, distant, absent, warm, loving, angry, cold,* etc. If you need some help getting started, consult the Relational Trait List on the next page. Even if you don't know them, these can also be people in the public arena (a politician) or generalizations ("artsy type" or "lawyers," for example).
2. Underline the three *best* traits.
3. Circle the three *worst* traits.

MY RELATIONAL PROFILE	
Positive Traits	Negative Traits

RELATIONAL TRAIT LIST

Accessible	Honest	Cautious	Afraid	Bright
Attentive	Loving	Supportive	Closed	Grumpy
Safe	Fair	Arrogant	Inflexible	Polite
Enthusiastic	Righteous	Crafty	Objective	Soothing
Loyal	Tolerant	Uninterested	Sensitive	Brave
Amiable	Boring	Beneficent	Harsh	Confident
Fragile	Jealous	Brash	Courageous	Persuasive
Creative	Wounding	Insensitive	Attacking	Trusting
Spiritual	Dependable	Stingy	Frank	Altruistic
Inviting	Connected	Open	Exact	Reliable
Intrusive	Cold	Impatient	Wise	Inappropriate
Mature	Agreeable	Blatant	Caring	Depressed
Sneaky	Sincere	Giving	Shallow	Unforgiving
Alert	Rough	Flexible	Playful	Stable
Critical	Thrifty	Firm	Dishonest	Dangerous
Shy	Tense	Immature	Spontaneous	Tactful
Kind	Bold	Virtuous	Grateful	Gentle
Responsible	Respectful	Assured	Brutal	Coarse
Silly	Tender	Humble	Available	Biased
Open-minded	Annoyed	Egotistical	Warm	Anxious
Intelligent	Stupid	Sweet	Resilient	Racist
Sexist	Angry	Compulsive	Family-oriented	Disciplined

Me-2-We Journey: Bubbly Delicious

Pick one person from your Easy bubble (page 8) and spend at least five minutes writing about this person in the space below (or write in your Me-2-We Journal).

Use one of the following prompts to help you:

One thing I love about this person is . . .
One thing I admire about this person is . . .
When I'm with this person, I feel . . .
My favorite memory with this person is . . .

_____

_____

_____

_____

_____

_____

_____

_____

_____

Dialogue and Write: The Good from Me, Myself, and I

Purpose: Practice using "I" messages, being mindful of the relationships around you, and being intentional in your positive relational acts.

Instructions:

1. Reach out to the person you identified on the previous page.

2. Share with them something you appreciate or admire about them using one of the following prompts:
   ~ "One thing I appreciate about you is . . ."
   ~ "One thing I admire in you is . . ."
   ~ "One thing I love about you is . . ."

   Elaborate on the *why* if you can. Do this unconditionally (without any expectations in return).

3. After, record below:
   ~ The person I shared with is _____.
   ~ I shared that I appreciated/admired/loved _____.
   ~ Their response/reaction was _____.
   ~ This made me feel _____.

Me-2-We Journey: Gas Bubbles

Pick one person from your Impossible bubble (page 9) and spend at least five minutes writing about this person in the space below (or write in your Me-2-We Journal).

Use one of the following prompts to help you:

One thing about this person that frustrates me is . . .

The story I tell myself about this person is . . .

I wish this person were more . . .

I wish my relationship with this person were . . .

Write: Test Your Relational Competency

Purpose: To identify your basic RC skills.

Instructions: Read each relational competency description and illustration and rate yourself from 1 to 10, with 10 as the highest score (i.e., I achieve that 100 percent of the time).

Don't worry! We imagine your score is not too impressive at the moment. But embedded in this chart are the skills you will learn throughout these sessions that you should already be familiar with from reading the book.

RELATIONAL COMPETENCY	DESCRIPTION	ILLUSTRATION	RATING (1–10)
Honoring boundaries	When I want to talk with someone, I check out in a warm voice tone whether they are available to listen at that time.	"Is now a good time to talk?"	
Honoring boundaries	When I want to talk and the person is not available at that time, I gently ask them to tell me when they are available and to let me know when that time comes.	"When would be a good time? And would you please come find me when the time comes?"	
Honoring boundaries	When someone wants to talk to me and I am not available at that time, I gently say when I can be available, and I initiate the conversation at the time I give them.	"I am not available right now, but I will be available in [minutes, hours, days]."	

RELATIONAL COMPETENCY	DESCRIPTION	ILLUSTRATION	RATING (1–10)
Honoring boundaries	When I am available, in a warm tone of voice I let them know I am available.	"I am available now."	
Relaxing defenses	Before I start talking or listening, I make eye contact and take three deep breaths to relax my eyes and express my intention.	(Makes eye contact, takes three breaths, and shares intention.) "My intention is to stay connected to you while I am talking." "My intention is to stay connected to you while I am listening."	
Expressing appreciations	When someone is available to listen to me, I express an appreciation for their availability.	"Thank you for being available to listen to what I want to say."	
Expressing appreciations	When someone says they are available to listen, I share an appreciation I have about them before I start talking.	"I have an appreciation for you that I want to share. When I see you do_____ [or hear you say_____], I really appreciate that."	
Speaker responsibility	When I speak with anyone, I start all my sentences with "I" rather than "you."	"Recently, I have been feeling_____, and I am curious about what you are thinking."	

RELATIONAL COMPETENCY	DESCRIPTION	ILLUSTRATION	RATING (1–10)
Speaker responsibility	When I am talking, I describe my thoughts and feelings rather than describing the person who is listening.	"Sometimes I think _____, and when I think that, I feel _____."	
Listener responsibility	When someone is talking to me and I get distracted or on overload, and can't listen anymore, I raise my hand and ask them to pause so I can mirror back what I heard so far, and then ask them to continue.	(Raises hand and says) "I would like to mirror what I have heard so far. If I got it, you said _____."	
Mirroring	After the person who is talking finishes their first few sentences, I mirror what I heard.	"Let me see if I am getting that. If I did, you said _____."	
Checking for accuracy	After I mirror what I heard the other person say, I check with them to see if I got it accurately.	"Did I get that?" or "Did I get you accurately?"	
Checking for accuracy	When I summarize what I heard, I check with the speaker whether my summary is accurate.	"Did I get everything you said?"	

RELATIONAL COMPETENCY	DESCRIPTION	ILLUSTRATION	RATING (1–10)
Checking for accuracy	After I share the feelings I see or imagine, I check to see if I got their feelings accurately.	"Is that the feeling?"	
Expressing curiosity	If they indicate I missed something, I ask them to send again the part I missed.	"Would you send again the part I missed?"	
Expressing curiosity	When the person I am listening to pauses, I ask them if they have more to say on the topic.	"Is there more about that?"	
Expressing curiosity	If the speaker says I did not get the feeling right, I ask them to share it again.	"Would you share your feeling with me again?"	
Expressing curiosity	After the feeling has been shared and confirmed, I ask if they have other feelings about that.	"Do you have other feelings about that?"	
Summarizing	When someone has finished speaking, I summarize what I heard.	"Let me see if I got everything you said. In summary, you said _____."	
Expressing validation	When someone has finished speaking, I validate the logic of what they are saying, whether I agree with them or not.	"You make sense, and what makes sense is that when you experienced _____ [event], you would have thought or felt _____."	

RELATIONAL COMPETENCY	DESCRIPTION	ILLUSTRATION	RATING (1-10)
Expressing empathy	When someone has finished speaking, I share with them the feelings I experienced their having or I imagine their feelings if they have not expressed them.	"Given all of that, I can see that you feel _____ [if their feelings are physically visible]." "I can imagine you might be feeling _____ [some version of mad, sad, glad, or scared]."	
Mirroring, accuracy check, and expressing curiosity	If the speaker has other feelings, I mirror the additional feelings and check for accuracy and completion.	"And you also feel _____. Did I get that accurately? Are there other feelings?"	
Expressing gratitude	If I am the listener, I express gratitude to the speaker at the end of a conversation for sharing their thoughts and feelings with me.	"Thanks for sharing your thoughts and feelings with me."	
Expressing gratitude	If I am the speaker, I express gratitude to the listener at the end of the conversation for listening to my thoughts and feelings.	"Thanks for listening."	
TOTAL SCORE (MAXIMUM 240)			

Write: My Relational Vision

Purpose: A vision turns energy away from past disappointments and toward a more hopeful future, the future we want to create. A vision gives direction to each decision and shapes each action. If you can imagine it, you can make it happen.

Overview: Imagining is almost as good as doing because a part of our brain does not distinguish between the two. (But imagining + doing is greater than either practice alone!) This exercise becomes the road map for your relational competency journey. It's shifting from what is lacking in your life to imagining its potential.

Instructions:

1. Spend five to ten minutes reading through the exercises and journal writing from this session.
2. Using the chart on page 11, write a series of statements that describe how you see yourself in relationship with others:
   ~ Write all sentences in the present tense, as if they already exist (even those that you are not yet doing).
   ~ Use "I" statements; short, descriptive sentences; and positive wording:

Positive Wording	Negative Wording
When I am in conflict, I seek to understand the other person.	I don't fight with others.

Examples:

I interact with people socially once a week.

I seek out people who are different from me and interest me.

Instead of reacting to people's differing opinions, I seek to understand their perspective.

I am a good listener.

I learn to share my thoughts and feelings in a way that does not diminish the other.

You can refer to the questions below to help generate some additional thoughts.

- How do I relate to Easy, Neutral, Challenging, and Impossible relationships?
- How curious am I about other people?
- How do I listen to others?
- How do I express my thoughts and feelings?
- How do I manage conflict?
- How do I nurture my relationships?
- How often do I see people socially?
- How proactive am I in seeking companionship?
- How do I seek other people's opinions that are different from my own?
- How do I handle negative thoughts and feelings about other people and myself?
- How do I generate positive thoughts and feelings about other people and myself?

MY RELATIONAL VISION
(Describe each behavior in positive, short sentences, in the present tense.)

Daily Do

- Write in your Me-2-We Journal.
- Read out loud or meditate on each sentence of your relationship vision. Feel free to edit, remove, and/or add as your vision grows. Visions should be fluid.
- Think daily about the relationships you have identified. Start noticing the interactions you have with people. What are you telling yourself inside? What are some of your assumptions about a particular person? How do you interact with them? Are you focusing on their negative traits? Are you self-conscious about what they are thinking about you?

Congratulations! You have started the RC journey.

Mirror, Mirror on the . . . Well, Everywhere

Review: Chapter 3

Introduction

Our SC Dialogue is a new way of talking that involves deep listening with intense curiosity and deep empathy. It creates a context in which no one involved is trying to change, control, or overpower anyone else. Instead, the goal is to see, hear, and value each other. SC Dialogue gives you a step-by-step guide to have conversations that are both safe and productive. Whether the topic is fun, like an appreciation, or something more serious and difficult, like sharing a frustration, Dialogue will ensure the conversation avoids negative triggers, elicits productive results, and keeps both parties in a relaxed, calm, and balanced state of mind.

The Old Way of Talking "Monologue"		The New Way of Talking "Dialogue"
Speaker and listener are both talking and neither is listening	→	Speaker and listener take turns talking and listening
One-way transaction	→	Two-way interaction
Creates inequality and distance	→	Creates equality and connection

SC Dialogue starts as a simple skill that consists of a speaker and listener following a three-step process that includes:

1. **Mirroring:** the listener accurately reflecting what they heard the speaker say.
2. **Validating:** the listener seeing the truth of the speaker's point of view, while retaining their own.
3. **Empathizing:** the listener accurately sharing how they experienced and/or imagined the emotions of the speaker as they are experiencing their world.

At the basic level, both parties take turns talking without judging, listening without criticizing, and connecting beyond differences. At the deepest level, Dialogue moves us away from transactional communication, which involves making deals, to transformational connecting, where we give without asking for something back. It begins as a skill to master but becomes a way of life and being.

If there is one thing to learn out of this entire manual, it is this: SC Dialogue is foundational and can transform your relationships and your life. This session will help you begin to practice the basic skills of Dialogue, with a focus on mirroring. We recommend you spend longer than a week on this section, until you are proficient in the basic mirroring stems.

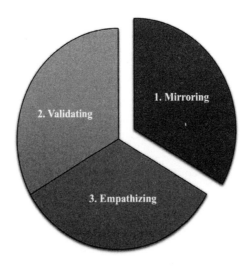

Read: Rewrite the You

Overview: Imagine someone says to you, "You are always late!" How does that make you feel? Do your defenses go up? Do you feel reactive inside?

Now imagine someone says to you, "I feel anxious and worried when you are running late because I don't know if you will show up in time for our meeting." How different does that feel to you?

"You" messages put the other on alert—stirring the fight, flight, or freeze response. "I" messages are easier to hear. They put the onus on the speaker's perspective and experience. Using "I" language is one of the "rules" that speakers follow when engaging in SC Dialogue.

 ## SPEAKER RESPONSIBILITY

- I feel . . .
- I am . . .
- I wish . . .
- I want . . .
- The story I tell myself . . .
  - ~ Uses "I" language
  - ~ Sends succinctly (one or two sentences at first).
  - ~ Focuses on one topic.
  - ~ Seeks to convey experience rather than opinions/judgments.
  - ~ Avoids phrases such as "you always" or "you never."
  - ~ Avoids all shaming, blaming, criticizing, belittling, or invalidating of the other person's perspective. This includes not only the words but the tone as well.

 ## LISTENER RESPONSIBILITY

- Makes eye contact.
- Is fully present to hear.

- Is open, curious, and nonjudgmental.
- Uses SC Dialogue sentence stems to help hear and understand the speaker's sharing.
- Gently puts up a hand if on overload and says, "Let me see if I got that so far . . ."
- Contains reactivity (desire to correct or question) and focuses on the speaker's message.

Write: Rewrite the You

Instructions: Read the "you" sentences on the left side. Using Speaker Responsibility, rewrite the sentence using "I" language and positive wording. Be creative! The idea is to start identifying how you might present things differently—especially when you disagree with someone or are frustrated. We filled in some blanks to help you get started.

Instead of . . .	Try . . .
"You never think about me!"	"I felt sad when you didn't give me a gift. The story I tell myself is that you don't care about me."
"You are always late! I can never rely on you!"	"When you are late, I feel frustrated and anxious about meeting our deadline."
"You never consider other people! The world doesn't revolve around you."	
"How can you feel that way?!"	
"You are [crazy, lazy, late, stupid, etc.]."	"I admire . . ."
"Are you listening to me?"	
"You really liked that movie?!"	
"How could you support that candidate?!"	

Read: Sentence Stems

Our SC Dialogue skill uses sentence stems to facilitate the three-step process. These consist of a sentence followed by a blank to be filled in by the speaker. Each sentence stem is designed to:

- create safety and relax defenses,
- regulate emotion,
- prevent negativity and polarization,
- deepen access to unspoken feelings and thoughts, and
- deepen the connection between speaker and listener.

In the beginning, sentence stems need to be memorized and used the way they are written. This helps eventually move us from structure to spontaneity, from skills practice to integration.

Read: Examples of Sentence Stems

- **Asking for an appointment:** The speaker verifies the availability of the listener.
  - ~ **Speaker:** "Is now a good time to talk about . . . ?"
- **Mirroring:** The listener focuses on repeating what the speaker has said.
  - ~ **Listener:** "Let me see if I got that. You said . . ."
- **Checking for accuracy:** The listener confirms with the speaker that the mirroring was accurate.
  - ~ **Listener:** "Did I get that?"
- **Showing curiosity:** The listener shows curiosity by asking for additional input.
  - ~ **Listener:** "Is there more about that?"
- **Summarizing:** When the speaker feels there is nothing further to say, the listener then summarizes the essence of what the speaker has said.
  - ~ **Listener:** "Let me see if I got all of that."
- **Validating:** The listener acknowledges the logic in the thought the speaker is expressing without necessarily agreeing.
  - ~ **Listener:** "You make sense, and what makes sense is . . ."
- **Empathizing:** The listener reflects or imagines the feeling that accompanies the speaker's perspective.
  - ~ **Listener:** "I can imagine that with all that, you might be feeling . . ."

Dialogue: Mirroring Stems

Let's start with mirroring. There are two ways to use mirroring:

Conversational Competency	Relational Competency
"À la carte" / Informal	Within a formal SC Dialogue process
Everyday and noncontentious conversations	For more challenging conversations
Often can just be mirroring	Uses all three steps of SC Dialogue

Instructions:

- This will require a practice partner.*
- Carve out thirty minutes to practice the mirroring stems.
- Decide who will be the first speaker and who will be the first listener.
- Each speaker can choose a sentence stem from the next page.
- Listener mirrors, checks for accuracy, and invites more. When there is no more, the listener provides a summary mirror and checks for accuracy. (Refer to Mirroring Sentence Stems on page 35.)
- After fifteen minutes, switch roles.

*If you do not have a practice partner, you can still practice as a listener using the sentence stems throughout your day. Practice as many stems as you can. If your boss gives you an assignment, mirror back the assignment, check for accuracy, and ask if there is more. If your friend shares a problem, do the same. Take the opportunity to be a listener, honing your listening and curiosity skills.

Practice: Conversation Starters

We will refer to this list throughout this workbook.

Easy Conversation Starters:

My favorite color is _____.

My favorite season is _____ because _____.

My favorite holiday is _____ because _____.

My favorite food/restaurant is _____.

I wish _____.

The superpower I wish I had is _____.

My favorite trip I've ever taken was _____ because _____.

I think the Beatles are better than the Rolling Stones (or vice versa) because _____.

I think cats are better than dogs (or vice versa) because _____.

I prefer coffee over tea (or vice versa) because _____.

I prefer sweet over savory (or vice versa) because _____.

If I were an animal, I would be a _____ because _____.

My least favorite chore is _____.

My favorite birthday was _____.

My favorite hobby is _____.

My favorite movie is _____.

My dream city is _____.

My dream house would be _____.

I find [name a sport or exercise] challenging because _____.

Something I have always wanted to learn (or try) is _____.

Something I like about my job is _____.

Something I would change about my job is _____.

My dream vacation is _____.

Something great that happened to me this week was _____.

I have a lot of respect for _____ because _____.

One thing people underestimate me for is _____.

Three words that would describe me are _____.

Deepening / More Intimate Conversation Starters (with closer friends, relatives):

Something that happened at work today was _____.

My best friend in elementary school was _____.

My perfect date was/would be _____.

A personal goal I have is _____.

I see myself in ten years doing _____.

My idea of a perfect day is _____.

A celebrity I had a crush on when I was growing up was _____.

I feel grateful for _____.

A positive childhood memory I have is _____.

I wish I were _____.

Growing up in my childhood home was _____.

I feel most happy when I'm with _____.

The most influential teacher I had growing up was _____.

My biggest insecurity is _____.

The best advice I've ever been given was _____.

My biggest fear in life is _____.

Boundaries I find most important are _____.

My favorite way to wake up is _____.

I would describe myself as _____.

I would like others to describe me as _____.

My biggest influence as a child was _____.

I want to work on _____ about myself.

If I could choose any career, I would be a _____.

The nicest thing anyone has done for me was _____.

I changed the most in my life during _____.

My guilty pleasure is _____.

One thing I would change about myself is _____.

One regret I have is _____.

Something that stresses me is _____.

Dialogue: Mirroring Sentence Stems

Speaker	Listener
Makes simple statement (sentence stem from page 35).	**Mirrors:** "Let me see if I got it. You said _____." **Checks for accuracy:** "Did I get it?"
Verifies accuracy: "Yes, you got it!" or "The part you got was _____. I also said _____."	Continues mirroring and checking for accuracy until speaker indicates, "You got it." **Shows curiosity:** "Is there more about that?"
Sends additional information (if desired) until there is no more.	**Summarizes:** "Let me see if I got all of that. You said _____." **Checks for accuracy:** "Is that a good summary?"
Thank each other for sharing/listening. Switch roles.	

Me-2-We Journey: To Hear and to Be Heard

Spend at least five minutes writing about your experiences with mirroring as both speaker and listener in the space below (or write in your Me-2-We Journal). Use the following prompts to guide your writing:

What it felt like to mirror . . .
What it felt like to be mirrored . . .

_____

_____

_____

_____

_____

_____

_____

_____

_____

_____

Read: Honing Our Listening Skills

How good of a listener are you? How good are you *really*? Does your mind wander a lot? When someone is sharing something with you, is your mind focusing more on your response rather than listening to their words? Or are you thinking of the errands you must do?

Our world is experiencing a crisis in listening as we try to drown each other out with our own opinionated voices, vying for ratings, subscribers, and clicks. Our attention spans are getting shorter and shorter. When not distracted but rather in a resting state, we still are lousy listeners. Indeed, we need to strengthen our listening muscles before listening becomes a lost art.

A popular saying attributed to the Dalai Lama is, "When you talk, you are only repeating what you already know. But if you listen, you may learn something new." And that is one of the goals in authentic listening: to learn something new (digging for "the golden nugget"). Other goals are to:

- be a witness to the other person (so they can be heard and valued);
- separate your "self" from their "self" and break your assumption that *they think, feel, and believe just like me*; and
- discover and see the sense in difference, and develop the ability for their differences to stand side by side with yours.

The goal is *not* to:

- solve someone's problem (although that could be an outcome if the other person is requesting help); or
- half-listen while preparing a legal brief to convince someone of their wrongness.

But listening is not only about hearing with the ears. We can also listen with our eyes (seeing a person's body language). We can listen with our hands (are they relaxed or fidgeting?) and with our heads (a compassionate nod or a scornful brow).

Practice: Honing Our Listening Skills

To help us with our listening skills, these daily practices can help us reduce stress and increase relaxation, quiet the inner chatter (so we can make room for the other), train our attention and awareness, curb reactivity and negativity, and increase our attention span:

1. Take five to ten minutes every morning to focus on your breathing and "empty" your mind of random thoughts. Make sure you are in a place with no distractions. You can focus on your breath (deep inhale through the nose for four counts; hold for seven counts; slow, deep exhale through pursed lips for eight counts). You can focus on a calming image, such as ocean waves crashing on the shore. Or you can repeat a word or sound over and over. If a thought comes up, recognize it, release it, and return to the breath, image, or sound.

2. Take five to ten minutes every day to take a walk outside, focusing on the senses—the sounds you hear, the sights you see, the feelings on your skin, the smells, and the tastes. If a thought (from the past, or things you need to do in the future) distracts you, let it go and observe the bark on the birch tree. If you think, *What should I make for dinner?* let it go and listen to the airplane flying overhead. Put all your attention in the here and now and the surrounding environment.

3. Take five to ten minutes to practice *niksen*, the Dutch word (and trend) that means "doing nothing." Do what you want, letting go of self- or other-imposed responsibilities. Doing nothing is unscripted and effortless.

Gradually build these daily practices to thirty to forty-five minutes daily, if possible. Other ideas to strengthen your listening muscle:

- Listen to audio podcasts.
- Listen to a song and focus on the lyrics. Play the song again and focus on one of the instruments. Play the song again and focus on another instrument. Then play it again, breathe deeply, and listen to the harmony of the voice and instruments together.

Me-2-We Journey: Hearing Ear to Ear

Spend at least five minutes writing down your experiences with listening. Use one of the prompts below or use stream of consciousness.

When focusing on listening, I discovered . . .
One thing I really heard for the first time was . . .
One thing I appreciated about listening is . . .
It is hard for me to . . .

_____

_____

_____

_____

_____

_____

_____

_____

_____

Write: Appreciations

Overview: Appreciations are a great way to: (1) practice mirroring, (2) create positive energy among people, and (3) move from a negative to a positive lens. How often do you feel appreciated at work? At home? With your friends? How often do you appreciate people in those environments? If your answer is "rarely" or "never," it's time to up your game and actively appreciate the people around you.

Instructions: Think of three people you interacted most with in the past week. Write down at least three things you appreciate about them. Use positive wording. It can be about a behavior or a trait.

Examples:

I appreciate how you make me coffee every morning.

I appreciate that you are ready to jump in when I need help at work.

I appreciate your philosophical mind and how you get me to think deeply about things.

I appreciate how artistic you are.

I appreciate how creative you are when you plan fun activities for the team.

Person 1	Person 2	Person 3

Dialogue: Mirroring an Appreciation

Overview: In this practice, we are adding two pieces to the mirroring step:

1. Making an appointment: This is an important step to honor boundaries. It moves us away from assuming someone is there for us whenever we want. We call this the "appointment-only rule," which insists that conversations (whether sharing something simple, such as an appreciation, or something more complex, such as a frustration) be by appointment only. It helps speakers honor boundaries and enables listeners to be fully available and present.

2. Deepening sentence stems: We also deepen our experience by using the sentence stems: "This makes me feel . . ." and "That feeling reminds me of a time in the past when . . ." It moves us from peripheral sharing to internal sharing, excavating layers underneath, which invites deeper connection.

Instructions:

1. You will need a practice partner for this exercise.
2. Follow the structure and use the sentence stems *precisely* as indicated in the Appreciation Dialogue on the next page.
3. When all the Dialogue steps are completed, switch roles and repeat the process.

MIRRORING AN APPRECIATION	
Speaker	**Listener**
Makes an appointment: "I would like to share an appreciation with you. Is now a good time?"	"I'm available now." (If not now, state when you will be available.)
Makes eye contact and takes three deep breaths in sync.	
"One thing I appreciate about you is _____."	**Mirrors:** "Let me see if I got it. You said _____." **Checks for accuracy:** "Did I get it?"
Verifies accuracy: "Yes, you got it." or "The part you got was _____. I also said _____."	Continues mirroring and checking for accuracy until speaker indicates "You got it." **Shows curiosity:** "Is there more about that?"
Deepens: "This makes me feel _____. And that feeling reminds me of a time in the past when _____."	Continues mirroring and checking for accuracy, and inviting more until there is no more.
	Summarizes: "Let me see if I got all of that. You said _____." **Checks for accuracy:** "Is that a good summary?"
Thank each other for sharing/listening. Switch roles.	

Me-2-We Journey: Bubbly Delicious x Two

Pick another person (different from last session) on your Easy list (page 8) and spend at least five minutes writing about this person in the space below (or in your Me-2-We Journal).

Use one of the following prompts to help you:

One thing I love about this person is . . .
One thing I admire about this person is. . . .
When I'm with this person, I feel . . .
My favorite memory with this person is. . . .

Read: Closing Thoughts

Initially, the SC Dialogue may feel artificial. With practice, it will become organic, seamless, and connecting. In the Dialogue, both partners cross a bridge into each other's worlds, motivated not only by the need to be heard and understood but also by the desire to hear and understand. The Dialogue ultimately says to the other, "I respect your otherness; I want to learn from it. And I want to share mine with you." In the process, we embrace our essential humanness—our differences yet fundamental connection. One of the greatest learnings of Dialogue is the discovery of two distinct worlds. Whenever two people are involved, there are always two realities. These realities will be different in small and large ways, no matter what. And the reality of the other person can be understood, accepted, valued, and even loved, but not made to be identical to our own.

Daily Do

- Share an appreciation for someone daily.
- Practice the mirroring sentence stems every day and throughout the day:
    - ~ while receiving instructions, requests, or tasks at work;
    - ~ when someone shares a concern or something personal with you;
    - ~ to echo questions your child asks;
    - ~ to repeat back ideas during meetings;
    - ~ when you feel reactive to something someone says.

You may not be able to use all the stems in an informal setting, but try to practice each of them separately if you cannot do them all at once.

1. **Boundaries:** "Is now a good time to talk about . . . ?"
2. **Mirroring:** "Let me see if I got that. You said . . ." or "If I got that, you said . . ."
3. **Deepening:** "This makes me feel . . ." and "That feeling reminds me of a time in the past when . . ."
4. **Checking for accuracy:** "Did I get that?"
5. **Expressing curiosity:** "Is there more about that?"
6. **Summarizing:** "If I got it all, you said . . . Is that a good summary?"

Everyday Examples:

"If I got it, you said you need this by 9:00 a.m. tomorrow. Did I get that? Is there more about that?"

"If I got it, you said pass the salt. Did I get that? Is there more about that?"

"If I got it, you said you had a rough weekend. Did I get that? Is there more about that?"

The goal is to practice these sentence stems until you no longer need to think about what's next. They roll off your tongue! You are strengthening the Dialogue muscles so when you really need them (i.e. you are feeling reactive about something someone said), you can employ these skills!

Proceed to the next session once you feel you have mastered the mirroring stems. As we move deeper into the sessions ahead, we will introduce the next two steps of Dialogue: validating and empathizing.

A Zero Negativity Lifestyle

Review: Chapter 5

Introduction

All thriving relationships have a nonnegotiable quality: safety. And safety and negativity are incompatible. That is why an essential skill in the SC process is achieving Zero Negativity (ZN).

Negativity is the major source of stress in all relationships. It is a dysfunctional interaction that seems endemic in humanity, often stemming from an intolerance to difference. Negativity stirs anxiety, inflaming debates and discussions into angry confrontations. We know this, yet it is all too easy to give in to our worst impulses when we feel threatened.

ZN essentially involves eliminating put-downs, name-calling, eye rolls, or any other form of shame, blame, or criticism of anyone and everyone. We understand that eliminating negativity in your interactions is not as easy as it sounds, but it is also a goal worthy of pursuing if you really want to build bridges and find common ground in your workplace, your community, your organizations, and your circle of acquaintances.

While ZN does mean refraining from all put-downs, negative comments and behaviors, it does not mean we cannot express our negative feelings or frustrations. Suppressed thoughts and feelings lead to passive-aggressive behavior or to the gradual dissolution of affection for one another. The flip side of ZN is learning to share negative feelings or frustrations in an intentional, responsible way.

The task may seem daunting, but the rewards are great. As negativity recedes, goodwill rushes in to fill the void. While we stepped up our positive yield in the previous session, in this session, we will decrease our negative output.

Write: ZN Pledge

Instructions: The first step in going ZN is to: (1) create an intention to remove negativity from your expressions, behaviors, and thoughts, and (2) create a gentle response when you experience negativity from someone else. Read, sign, and date the pledge below. You will learn more about signals and the Reconnecting process in this session.

I understand that "negativity" is any interaction that ruptures my connection with another person, whether intentional or accidental.

I pledge to make all of my relationships and conversations zones of Zero Negativity for the next sixty days by omitting from all my interactions to the best of my ability any words, tones, behaviors, or body language that could be interpreted as a put-down.

If I experience a negative reaction from someone and feel threatened, I will immediately send a gentle signal ("Bing," "Ouch," "Wow," "Oops!") to communicate that I have experienced a put-down and then, when possible, use the Reconnecting process to restore safety and to connect.

Signed _____

Date _____

Write: Coming Up with a Signal

Overview: Many of us assume that those who say negative things to us know we're upset (this is that self-absorption phenomenon—assuming that people think, feel, and act like me, or believing that they should!). Some people lack the ability to read the reactions of those they offend. Or they might think we're "too sensitive" (ouch!). Some comments were intended in another way but land differently. For example, text messages that are deprived of facial expressions and tone are often interpreted for their literal meaning only. Not only have you probably experienced this, but you most likely (unknowingly and unintentionally, of course) have done this to others.

Instead of stomping in silence, swearing the relationship off, or escalating with a war of words, in the SC process, we offer a gentle signal to other people, letting them know when their comment or behavior landed negatively (a put-down). The idea for a gentle signal is having the opportunity to contain and reframe our responses to keep negativity at bay.

Instructions: With your practice partner, discuss a signal that you could use when you experience negativity. You could share the same signal or create your own. If you do not have a practice partner, come up with a signal that you can still use to let people know when you have experienced something negative from them (a put-down). For people who are not familiar with the SC process, having a short elaboration using "I" language after the signal is helpful. Please review the examples below.

Examples of Signals: "Ouch." "Wow." "Oops." "Bing."

My signal with my practice partner: _____

My practice partner's signal: _____

My signal for others: _____

Examples of Elaborations:

"I don't think you meant to be hurtful, but I felt criticized when you said . . ."

"I felt that was a zinger."

"I experienced that as a little harsh."

"That felt a bit disparaging to me."

"Could you reframe that?"

Tips: Going Zero Negative

1. **Start with an achievable goal:** We remind people to start with small goals. For couples taking our workshop, we ask them to first pledge to ZN for the remainder of our weekend time together. For others, we encourage taking a sixty-day ZN Challenge. For others still, even a twenty-four-hour commitment can be a stretch and all they can commit to at that time. Once you build up small successes, you can commit to longer periods of time.

2. **Self-reflect:** Keep in mind that the goal is not to repress the feelings behind our negative thoughts and behaviors—that would only add to our store of pent-up emotions—but rather to recognize them and make a change. One of the best ways to start solving a relationship problem is to look at your own contribution: *Here I am again, having critical thoughts about _____. What does this say about me? What am I doing or not doing right now that is feeding my negative attitude? What is my fear behind this feeling?* In time, you'll begin to notice all the ways you were being critical—making jokes at others' expense, speaking negatively about them to others, ruminating passive-aggressive thoughts. This awareness itself can motivate change.

3. **Centering strategies:** Develop strategies to help ground yourself that you can employ at any given moment. For example, if you typically dread attending team meetings, ask yourself, *What am I prepared to leave outside this meeting room in order to be fully present?* or listen to that sonata that evokes a sense of oneness before stepping into the conference room. If you struggle with social anxiety, use sensory grounding techniques, such as walking barefoot in the grass, using a fidget gadget, or sucking on a sour candy to move from the thoughts to the sensations. Focus on the present moment by slowly naming things you can see, touch, feel, taste, and hear.

Me-2-We Journey: A Different Kind of Mirror

Pick one person from your Challenging or Impossible bubble (page 9). Spend a few minutes thinking about the negativity you feel toward them. Is there something about this person you can use to learn something about yourself? Spend at least five minutes writing down your thoughts in the space below (or use your Me-2-We Journal).

Use one of the following prompts to help you:

What does this negativity say about me?

What am I doing or not doing right now that is feeding my negative attitude?

What is my fear behind this feeling?

What is my wish underneath this feeling?

Why do I care enough to have attached feelings around them?

Is there something about this person that is just like me?

Does this person—or the way they make me feel—remind me of someone else?

Write: A New Script on My Negative Messages

Overview: Many of us harp on the negative. It could even be negative things about us *(I'm too old! I'll never be in a relationship. No one likes me. I'm incompetent/unlovable/a basket case).* And the more negatively we think, the more negative we feel, and before long we find ourselves jumping down the rabbit hole, spiraling through a dark tunnel, echoing negative messages about ourselves or others. This is our script or modus operandi. A practice to help move away from negativity is akin to fishing instructions: catch it, reel it in, and recast.

These negative messages stem from a variety of factors (all relational), including societal messages, cultural influences, childhood experiences, religious tenets, and the influence of teachers and friends. We might have assumptions about gender, race, class, or the way a person looks. We might be our own worst critic. Remember, though, these are not facts. They are beliefs influenced by the messages we received. As part of going ZN, we let go of judgment and move into acceptance. We detach ourselves from the negative feelings surrounding a core belief.

Instructions: During the next week, catch yourself with your negative thoughts. It could be about yourself or others. Using the chart on the next page, write down these messages in the left column. In the right column, rewrite the script. Think about how you can turn that into a goal, an acceptance, or an admiring trait.

Examples:

Instead of "Harry is so critical," try "He has a discerning eye for mistakes."
Instead of "I am old," try "I am wise."
Instead of "I'm out of shape," try "I'm going to walk ten minutes a day."
Instead of "I'm not good enough," try "I'm good enough and I can be better."

REWRITING THE SCRIPT The Put-Downs	
Instead of . . .	**Try . . .**

Write: A New Script on My Frustrations

Purpose: To translate your frustrations into desires.

Overview: Many times, underneath a complaint or a frustration about someone is a wish in disguise. For example, if your son is messy and you find yourself regularly yelling at him about his sloppiness, your wish might be that he keeps his room clean on a regular basis without being reminded. Yes, we realize this might be wishful thinking, but the purpose of this exercise is to practice learning how to translate our frustrations into ways that are responsible and accessible for the other to hear (for example, moving from "you" messages to "I" messages).

Instructions: During the next week, recognize when you feel frustrated. It could be about yourself or others. Using the chart on the next page, write down these frustrations or complaints in the first column. In the second column, write down the feeling underneath the frustration or complaint. In the third column, rewrite the script! Think about the wish underneath the frustration or complaint and the global desire that would remove the frustration.

REWRITING THE SCRIPT
The Wish under the Complaint or Frustration

Frustration or Complaint	Feelings	Desire
I feel frustrated when...	This makes me feel...	I wish...
Sally is late to work.	angry that I have to pick up her slack.	Sally was on time.

Read: The Reconnecting Process

Sometimes a simple signal is enough to turn around a put-down, especially for nonfamilial relationships. But for more intimate relationships (your spouse, family members, friends), sometimes the put-down opens a sore and leaves us feeling deeply hurt, vulnerable, or angry. And more than just a signal is needed to help reconnect the relationship. To review, here are some things to help you reconnect with others after experiencing a put-down:

1. Ask for a do-over. Take a time-out from the conversation for a little mental-health break, start over, and try reframing the conversation in a more positive manner. "This conversation isn't working for either of us. Let's try this again."

2. Use mirroring and suggest language that is more positive and not hurtful. "I hear you are not happy with my performance. Can you suggest some ways that I can be more productive?"

3. Offer a way to reconnect. "Why don't we take a break, have a cup of coffee somewhere, and take turns listening to each other's perspective on this?"

4. Have a SC Dialogue about the feelings that came up. "When I heard I wasn't invited, I felt hurt. And I wonder if I did something to upset you."

5. Offer a gift or change in behavior. It might include a sincere apology from each of you, offering each other three appreciations, a kind note, an exchange of gifts, having a meal together, or any combination of the above.

And because we are all different, what might work for some will not work for others. For me (Helen), I need an apology and an appreciation. For me (Harville), I want a do-over and a lottery card (that wins!).

Write: If at First I Don't Succeed

Instructions: Think about recent put-downs you experienced from others. Consider what would have worked to help you reconnect with that person. It might be several things or one thing, or it might be one thing that occurs with different people.

 Tips:

1. If you have a practice partner, use Dialogue to share a recent put-down experience and what would have helped to reconnect.
2. For those who are not familiar with this process, when someone experiences a put-down from you, ask them, "What can I do to help fix that?" and offer some examples (apologize, resend the message, join them for a walk, have a coffee break together).
3. What counteracts a put-down for me is . . .

_____

_____

_____

_____

_____

_____

_____

Write: Sixty Days of Zero Negativity

Instructions: Monitor your negativity for the next sixty days. At the end of each day, spend a few minutes reviewing your experiences, behaviors, and thoughts, and rate your ZN success. Use the calendar on the next page or buy your own calendar that is solely for this practice.

If you feel you went throughout the day without being negative, then give yourself a smiley face on the calendar for that day. If you felt that you had negative thoughts or behaviors but quickly reconnected or adjusted, give yourself a smiley face. If you felt you had negative thoughts or behaviors and didn't reconnect, give yourself a frowning face and make a pledge to do better tomorrow. The goal is to be conscious of our negativity and aim for a ZN lifestyle!

Monday	Tuesday	Wednesday	Thursday	Friday	Saturday	Sunday

Write: The Space-Between

Overview: The Space-Between is the intangible space between you and others. The more negative behaviors and qualities in the Space-Between, the greater the chance for conflict and rupture. As you begin to remove negativity from your relationships, it is important to intentionally acknowledge the negative qualities that you contribute to your Space-Between in your relationships.

Instructions: Consider your relationships (home, work, classroom, house of worship, etc.). Using negative descriptors (examples below), describe your experience of the Space-Between in that relational ecosystem to complete the sentences below.

Purpose: To become aware of your contribution to the Space-Between.

1. The negative qualities that describe the Space-Between me and my relationships include: _____

2. The negative qualities I bring to this Space-Between are: _____
_____

3. The negative behaviors I bring to this Space-Between are: _____
_____

NEGATIVE DESCRIPTORS OF THE SPACE-BETWEEN (EXAMPLES)	
Criticism	Shame
Sarcasm	Competition
Passive-aggressive behavior	Grudges
Assumptions	Dishonesty
Righteousness	Ignoring
Devaluing	Teasing

Draw: The Space-Between

Instructions: Consider all your relationships (home, work, classroom, house of worship, etc.) and draw your ideal experience of the Space-Between.

Daily Do

- Choose a conversation starter from page 37 and have a Dialogue with your practicing partner.
- Share an appreciation with someone new.
- Monitor your ZN by using a calendar.
- Write in your Me-2-We Journal.
- Read out loud or meditate on each sentence of your relational vision.
- Practice the mirroring sentence stems throughout the day every day.
- Practice emptying your mind by meditating, walking outside and focusing on your senses, and doing nothing (*niksen*).

Proceed to the next session once you feel you have at least seven days straight of ZN and you feel it is becoming easier to recognize your negativity.

I Get You

Review: Chapter 4

Introduction

Validation and empathy are the second and third (and final) steps of the SC Dialogue. After mirroring accurately until there is "no more," seeing the sense in the speaker's experience should be relatively easy. Validation merely recognizes that the other person makes sense, given their experience and interpretation. It lets go of absolute truths and allows their world to stand equally with yours.

Think of the ancient parable of the blind men and an elephant. Each man describes a different part of the elephant—all of which are true in their depiction but seem contradictory to one another. Or think of two people sitting across from each looking at a number on the table between them. One sees the number 6 and the other sees the number 9. Both are right from where they are sitting!

Validation is a reminder that you don't have to agree with the speaker's view, but that, from their

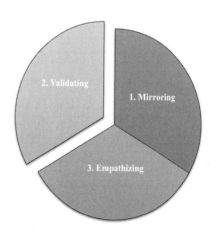

perspective, they make sense. This can be difficult for many because they incorrectly assume that validating means "I agree." Validation begins to break the assumption that you must be like me. Validation instead says that you are you, which is different from me, and that's okay.

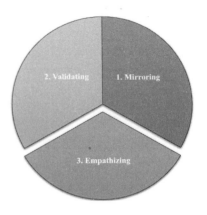

Empathy is an exercise in "feeling with" the other (the speaker) and imagining what their world feels like given their experience. It is the ability to understand and relate to the feelings and perspectives of others, while being able to maintain one's separate self, participating in the other's interior world, while simultaneously holding on to one's distinctive world. Many of us, however, have lost our ability to empathize due to our self-absorption, the state of isolation we inhabit when we experience the anxiety of early ruptured connections. But empathy can be learned.

Dialogue provides the structure to mature our validation and empathy skills. Empathy comes after the validation piece of Dialogue because when we *really* listen and *really* understand, we can connect the dots, see the other as another (not as an extension of the self), and seamlessly imagine (or feel) the emotions behind the experience. Throughout Dialogue, listeners listen for the emotions the speaker is experiencing. If the emotions are not visible, the listener tries to imagine or intuit how the speaker must feel, given the content they just communicated.

There are two types of empathy: cognitive and participatory. Cognitive empathy is the ability to recognize, understand, and articulate another's emotions ("Given what you said, I imagine you might be feeling . . ."). Participatory empathy is being attuned to (feeling with) the other's experience, while maintaining our own. This second level of empathy communicates, "I understand what you understand because I am experiencing what you are experiencing, although I remain myself." Both cognitive and participatory empathy communicate to the speaker a respect for their feelings and perspective, even if the listener doesn't share the same feelings or point of view. This kind of empathic attunement is ultimately the goal in a SC Dialogue. Mirroring says, "I hear you." Validating says, "I respect you." And empathy says, "I feel you."

In this session, we will practice validating and cultivating empathy through understanding the role of stories and curiosity.

Dialogue: Peeling Back the Layers

Instructions:

1. You will need a practice partner for this Dialogue.
2. Decide who will be the first speaker and who will be the listener.
3. Choose a conversation starter from page 37.
4. Follow the structure and use the sentence stems as indicated on the next page, paying attention to the deepening stems listed.
5. As the speaker shares, add at least one of these sentence stems to deepen the experience:
   a. "When I experience(d) _____, I feel/felt _____."
   b. "What I am afraid of is _____."
   c. "When I feel/felt that, I react(ed) by _____."
   d. "What this feeling reminds me of is _____."
6. Continue the full SC Dialogue experience (validation and empathy). When listeners are empathizing, remember feelings can be expressed in one word. For example, *happy, angry, confused, sad, cherished*. Remember to check for accuracy of the feelings. ("Are those feelings accurate?")
7. When all the SC Dialogue steps are completed, switch roles and repeat the process.

DIALOGUE: DEEPENING STEMS PRACTICE One-Page Overview	
Makes (and agrees to) an appointment.	
Makes eye contact and takes three deep breaths in sync.	
Shares an appreciation.	Mirrors appreciation and checks for accuracy.
Shares a conversation starter. Listens to mirror and verifies accuracy.	Mirrors, checks for accuracy, and invites more.
Deepens the share using one or more of these statements. "When I experience(d) _____ I feel/felt _____." "What I am afraid of is _____." "When I feel/felt that, I react(ed) by _____." "What this feeling reminds me of is _____."	Continues mirroring, checking for accuracy, and inviting more.
Speaker continues deepening until there is no more. Listener continues mirroring, checking for accuracy, and inviting more until there is no more.	
Listens to and confirms the summary. If something was missed, resend that part again.	Summarizes and checks for accuracy.
Listens to and confirms validation.	Validates and checks for accuracy.
Listens to and confirms feelings.	Empathizes and checks for accuracy.
Gives each other a handshake or high five, or with an intimate partner gives each other a one-minute hug. Expresses gratitude to each other for sharing/listening. Switches roles.	

Tips: Feeling with Others

Empathy is:

- judgment-free. The other's feelings are valid given their experience and perspective—even if you would feel differently.
- being present for—and witness to—someone else's (joyful, painful, frightening, angry, etc.) experience. Remember, we are striving to see, hear, and value (and to be seen, heard, and valued).

Empathy is not:

- imagining how the listener would feel if the listener was in the speaker's shoes. It's imagining what the speaker is feeling while in the speaker's shoes.
- "fixing" or "minimizing" the emotions of the speaker. Statements like, "You'll feel better" or "This, too, shall pass" devalue the speaker's experience.
- comparing experiences or hijacking their story. For example, saying, "I imagine you feel hurt because the same thing happened to me," or "I know just how you feel!" immediately brings the "I" (the listener) into the picture when it should be about "you" (the speaker).

Read: Discovering My Story

Overview: When we meet another, our past is alive and well in the present, influencing our assumptions, behaviors, expectations, feelings, and responses. We are shaped by the pains and frustrations, the joys and celebrations from the past. We move in our world of present-day relationships with these recorded monologues, often fearful of difference and with a compulsive need to be right. All these memories of past experiences lie in the Space-Between. And if those things remain unconscious, it prevents an authentic meeting between I and Thou.

It is important to connect the past with the present for two reasons: (1) to provide insight to the sharer (speaker), and (2) to invite empathy to the witness (listener). Deepening our sharing with sentence stems invites us to break the unconscious grip of the past on the present, to make sense of the behaviors and feelings, and to participate via empathy of the other. It also means being vulnerable, but that is where depth and authenticity lie. When we can excavate the feelings underneath the frustration and the memories under the feelings, then we can connect the dots to our experiences. And it is not just negative feelings and experiences but positive ones as well. Positive memories are those when a present behavior touches the heart just right. These past experiences shaped us into the "I that I am."

In the next couple of exercises, we invite you to explore the past, but it is important to tread lightly. The purpose is not to dwell or get stuck there but to discover your story and how it influences your current relationships. If you were the youngest in a family of six, you might have experienced being left out by the older siblings—a feeling that is poignant when you see some people at work go out to lunch together. Or perhaps you were criticized by your father (as his way of pushing you to be your best) and now find that a sarcastic joke by a friend hurts a little too much (even though you cognitively can understand "it was just a joke"). Once we understand these early triggers, the emotional charge dissipates, and we are freer to move into new behaviors and acceptance. We inhale the knowledge of our pasts and exhale the actions of our futures.

Caution: If, at any point, you are experiencing any strong emotions or memories, stop and seek professional help (see Additional Resources in the back of this workbook).

Me-2-We Journey: Once Upon a Time

Close your eyes, take a deep breath, and think about your early life and/or childhood home. Briefly recall positive experiences with your parents, friends, siblings, classmates, etc. Then use one of those positive memories to write on the next page (or in your Me-2-We Journal), including the corresponding feeling that went with the experience.

Alternatively, you can draw a picture of the experience.

Me-2-We Journey: Once Upon a Time

Close your eyes, take a deep breath, and think about your early life and/or childhood home. Briefly recall frustrations you experienced with your parents, friends, siblings, classmates, etc. Then choose one of the mild frustrations and write about it on the next page (or in your Me-2-We Journal), including the corresponding feeling that went with the experience.

Alternatively, you can draw a picture of the experience.

Write: My Adult Relational Need

Overview: Our relationship needs appear in clever disguises. There may be a pattern or a regularity. For example, we may need to arrive at the airport hours in advance because we're triggered by memories of late or chaotic travel in our youth. Or our need to be a little messy rebels against the controlling environment of our early childhood years. Understanding and sharing what has occurred in our lives to trigger a need is a pathway to validation and empathy—the key elements for safety and connection.

Instructions: Think about the need you experience(d) in your most significant relationships. This need could apply to a significant other, an ex, or a close family member. Study the list below and circle one of the needs that best reflects those experiences. If needed, you may expand with notes in the space provided.

THE RELATIONSHIP NEED I EXPERIENCE(D)	
To be free to do what I want to do with my time	To experience interest in what I am talking about
To be trusted by others for my thinking and my decisions	To be asked for my opinion on subjects being discussed
To have my emotional and physical boundaries honored when I set them	To be included when plans are being made
To experience recognition and appreciation for my perspective	To experience others being curious about my experiences in life
To experience what I do being valued by others	To be valued for who I am as well as what I do

Write: The Past Challenge

Overview: Associating a past challenge or experience with a current relationship need is a powerful way of continuing to understand our stories. Our experiences with people in the past shape the behavior and quality of our relationships in the present.

Instructions: Study the list below and circle the past challenge that best describes what triggered the need you identified on the previous page. If needed, you may expand with notes in the space provided.

THE PAST CHALLENGE THAT TRIGGERED MY NEED	
Experiencing being controlled by others	Feeling invisible, unseen, and unvalued
Being told what to think and how to express my thoughts	Feeling abandoned and alone
Being told what and how to feel	Experiencing myself as insignificant
Experiencing my thoughts and feelings as not important to others	Receiving no support for what I thought and felt
Being told what to do and how to do it	Feeling that what I wanted and liked was uninteresting to others

Dialogue: The Relationship Need Dialogue

Overview: The Relationship Need Dialogue is a structured guide for creating connection instead of rupture when we articulate our needs, and it leads to empathy and respect for one another—our intimate partners, family members, peers, and colleagues.

Instructions:

1. You will need a practice partner for this Dialogue.
2. Use the exercise on the previous pages to prepare for this Dialogue.
3. Decide who will be the first speaker and who will be the listener.
4. Follow the structure and use the sentence stems precisely as indicated.

DIALOGUE: SHARING A RELATIONAL NEED

Speaker	Listener
Makes an appointment: "I would like to have a Dialogue about a relationship need I have [at home, at work, or in my community]. Is now a good time?"	"I'm available now." *(If not now, state when you will be available.)*
Makes eye contact and takes three deep breaths in sync.	
Shares an appreciation: "Before I start, I would like to share an appreciation. I appreciate that you _____ [shares something special or important about the listener]."	**Mirrors:** "Let me see if I got it. You appreciate that I _____." **Checks for accuracy:** "Did I get it?"

DIALOGUE: SHARING A RELATIONAL NEED	
Speaker	Listener
Verifies accuracy: "Yes, you got it" or "The part you got was _____. I also said _____."	**Shows gratitude:** "Thank you for sharing that."
Shares a relational need: "I'd like to tell you about a need I have [or had] in my relationship [at home, at work, or in my community]. This need is _____ [circled on page 87]."	**Mirrors and checks for accuracy:** "Let me see if I got that. You said _____. Did I get that?"
Verifies accuracy: "Yes, you got it." or "Yes, and I also said _____."	**Continues mirroring and checking for accuracy** until speaker indicates, "You got it." **Shows curiosity:** "Is there more you'd like to say about this relationship need?"
Deepens: "This relationship need reminds me of a challenge I had in my past [recent or distant], which is _____ [the past challenge circled on page 89]."	**Continues mirroring and checking for accuracy:** "Let me see if I've got it. The relationship need you have reminds you of a past challenge, which is _____. Did I get it?" **Invites more:** "Is there more about that?"

DIALOGUE: SHARING A RELATIONAL NEED	
Speaker	**Listener**
"When I remember this, it makes me feel _____ [sensations, feelings, emotions]."	**Mirrors and checks for accuracy:** "Let me see if I've got that. When you remember this past challenge, you feel _____. Did I get that?"
Speaker continues deepening until there is no more. Listener continues mirroring, checking for accuracy, and inviting more until there is no more.	
Listens to and confirms the summary. If something was missed, resend that part again.	**Summarizes:** "Let me see if I got all of that. You are experiencing a need in your relationships [at home, work, or in community], which is _____. This relationship need reminds you of _____ [challenge in the past]. And it makes you feel _____." **Checks for accuracy:** "Is that a good summary?"
Confirms the validation. If anything was not validated, asks to send that part again.	**Validates:** "You make sense! What makes sense is that the relationship need you have, which is _____, reminds you of _____. And it makes sense that this memory causes you to feel _____." **Checks for accuracy:** "Is that a good validation?"

DIALOGUE: SHARING A RELATIONAL NEED

Speaker	Listener
Listens to and confirms empathy: "Yes." or "Yes, I'd also feel _____."	**Expresses empathy:** "I can imagine that if this relationship need was met by _____ [new actions or behaviors], you would feel _____ [glad, happy, fulfilled, joyful, etc.]." **Checks for accuracy:** "Is that your feeling? Are there other feelings?"

Give each other a handshake or high five,

or with an intimate partner give each other a one-minute hug.

Expresses gratitude to each other for sharing/listening. Switches roles.

Read: Their Story

Overview: Now that you have explored some of your story and how that might impact your current relationships, it is time to think about how everyone has a story. What we see and think of people can be just a piece of their larger narrative.

You might not know their story, but there is a narrative that explains their presentational self (the self that is portrayed to the world). Maybe someone who is critical experienced a critical father and never felt accepted for who they are. Or someone who shows little emotion lost their mom to cancer when they were five. Perhaps rejection and bullying by school peers created prejudices. It might be that the person in the cubicle next to you has an autoimmune disease they battle daily.

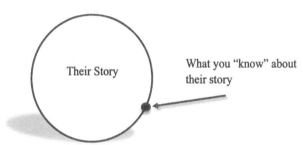

The first step in discovering another's story is unknowing someone, letting go of your assumptions, understanding that there are some things you do not know (nor will you ever know) about someone else.

The second step is becoming curious. Why is a person acting that way? What is their motivation or intention? What is the *more* (the feelings, fears, past influences) underneath? Curiosity is antithetical to judgment and criticism. The sentence stem "Is there more about that?" invites listeners to move from judgment to curiosity.

As a couple, we learned early on that it was a mistake to merely assume we knew what each of us needed from the other. We needed to take the time to be curious, ask questions, listen, and understand what we wanted from each other. The same holds true in all relationships.

We realize it can be challenging to be empathic toward someone if you perceive them as hurting you, vengeful, or hateful (especially if they are igniting your own triggers). But everyone has a story. Everyone has some sort of internal battle or a fear of being unseen, unheard, or unvaluable. Even the most self-absorbed people present a facade to hide a deep fear of rejection.

Me-2-We Journey: The Stories I Make Up

Pick one person in your Challenging or Impossible bubble (page 9) and spend at least five minutes writing about the assumptions you have of this person and the questions you would ask to get to know them better. Write in the space below (or in your Me-2-We Journal).

Use one of the following prompts to help you:

Assumptions I have about this person are . . .

If I could ask questions about this person, I would ask . . .

The story I tell myself about this person is . . .

Maybe this person is . . .

_____

_____

_____

_____

_____

_____

_____

_____

_____

_____

_____

Read: The Whys of Empathy

Empathy invites an inner excavation of hidden thoughts and feelings that makes it safe to bring them to the surface. It allows the speaker to formulate, express, and share ideas and feelings that might not have been realized or expressed ever before. Empathy can help us truly hear one another, because when there is receptivity and a safe space, words will flow. Unless we excavate our hidden stories into a conscious light, they will continue sabotaging our relationships.

Empathy ultimately motivates speakers to stretch beyond their comfort zone in the service of the other. It requires a great deal of courage for listeners to open themselves to truly receive. The give-and-take that is experienced in reciprocity can narrow the Space-Between individuals with differences and fill the gaps that have separated them.

Daily Do

- Continue Dialoguing with your practice partner using a conversation starter from page 37.
- Share an appreciation with someone new.
- Monitor your ZN using a calendar.
- Write in your Me-2-We Journal.
- Read out loud or meditate on each sentence of your relational vision.
- Practice the mirroring sentence stems every day and throughout the day.
- Practice emptying your mind by meditating, walking outside and focusing on your senses, and doing nothing (*niksen*).
- Pay attention to the assumptions you make about the people around you—even a stranger walking past you on the street.
- Be curious about something anyone shares with you—from the mundane to the exceptional—by mirroring and inviting more ("Is there more about that?" or "I would love to hear more about that!").

Proceed to the next session once you feel a shift from judgment to curiosity and you begin connecting your story on how the past influences the present.

The Practice of Affirmations

Review: Chapter 6

Introduction

More than ever, we need to tap into our emotional reservoir and jump-start those positive, feel-good neurochemicals that strengthen our resilience. Instead of a vicious cycle in which some of us may find ourselves, we need to create a virtuous cycle. The more we intentionally focus on the good, the more good there will be on which to focus.

When we first embraced ZN as a way to save our marriage, an interesting thing happened. Silence. Painful silence. We had been so negative with each other that when we removed the criticism, blame, and shame in the Space-Between, there was nothing left! We had been so preoccupied with knocking the other one down, we now needed a pathway to build each other up, to infuse the Space-Between with positive energy. With that in mind, we added Affirmation as the fourth skill of the SC process. This turned out to be essential. It completed the steps that help create, restore, and sustain connection, even with those who hold differing views and opinions.

Affirmation speaks directly to all three desires (to be seen, heard, and valued). It is unconditional acceptance of the other and the celebration of difference. Forms of affirmations include appreciation, recognition, positive valuation, and validation—both given and received. In this session we will deepen the Affirmation process of appreciation, which we have mentioned before, and will add other affirming actions to our relational competency inventory.

Dialogue: The 7 A's

The Affirmation process includes seven practices. With your practice partner, decide who is going first, and do the following. Then switch roles.

1. Ask for an appointment to share the 7 A's.
2. Make eye contact and take three deep breaths in sync.
3. Say slowly and out loud the sentences below, putting emphasis on the A-words.

    I *acknowledge* you.

    I *accept* you.

    I *appreciate* you.

    I *admire* you.

    I *affirm* you.

    I *advocate* you.

    I *adore* you as you are.

    Thank you for the gift of you!
4. The listener sits and takes it all in. The listener does not mirror. Then the listener becomes the speaker.

Me-2-We Journey: Warm and Fuzzy

Spend a few minutes thinking about the kinds of appreciations you have given to people over the course of this journey. Envision their faces and hear their responses. Now spend at least five minutes writing in the space below (or in your Me-2-We Journal) how it felt to give appreciations. Use at least one of the prompts below to assist you:

One thing I learned about myself from giving appreciations is . . .

What I love about giving appreciations is . . .

The best response from giving an appreciation was . . .

Giving appreciations daily helped me . . .

Read: Appreciations Take Two

Appreciations take place in the interactive space, in the Space-Between. Thus, when we share appreciations with another, we are participating in the oscillating energy that is the substance of all that is in the universe, including ourselves.

There are different levels of appreciations. *Simple* appreciations include quick gestures, such as a smile with a "thank you, I appreciate that" when someone opens a door or "I really appreciate how you greet Huxley every morning with your contagious and genuine smile!" to your son's bus driver. There might be a momentary shift in both the giver and the receiver.

There are also *eloquent* appreciations that might be shared with, for example, a colleague surrounded by witnesses at the beginning of a work meeting. An eloquent appreciation might look like this: "Mark, I have been looking over the financial plan you put together for our company, and I appreciate your careful attention to detail. I feel confident in the numbers, and I feel so fortunate having you on our financial team." These become a little more impactful—for the giver, the receiver, and even the witnesses. Positive feelings may radiate outward and stick around for longer than just a moment.

Then there are *deep* appreciations that are reserved for closer relationships. They carve out time from our busy lives to share an appreciation and unpack some of the layers beneath. These are the ones that, with repetition, invite new neural pathways for both the giver and the recipient. These appreciations are very different, neurochemical-producing experiences. They are transformational.

Write: Appreciations Take Two

Instructions: Choose someone in your Easy bubble (page 8) and share a *deep* appreciation this week via a handwritten note. Use the prompts below:

I appreciate when you . . .
When you do that, I feel . . .
And it reminds me of when . . .
Thank you for that gift!

Dialogue: Affirmations Dialogue

Instructions: Spend a few minutes thinking about a time in the past that made you feel heard, seen, and valued (at home, work, or in your community). Then, with your practice partner, using the Affirmations Dialogue (all three steps), share the memory.

Prompts for Speaker:

- "I would like to have a Dialogue about something that made me feel seen and valued. Is now a good time?"
- "I felt seen and valued as a person when [describe the behavior]."
- "When I experienced that, I felt _____."
- "That feeling reminds me of _____."

Prompts for Listener:

- Mirrors, checks for accuracy, and invites more throughout.
- When there is no more:
  - ~ Summarizes (and checks for accuracy)
  - ~ Validates (and checks for accuracy)
  - ~ Empathizes (and checks for accuracy)

Read: What a Surprise!

Many people give each other presents on special occasions like birthdays and Hanukkah. These gifts are so customary that they are almost taken for granted. Although the presents may be enjoyed, they don't carry the same emotional impact as a present that is given as a total surprise. Surprises are the hot sauce of relationships and the protection against the boredom and flatness of habituation. Our neuronal systems are wired from birth to respond both to familiarity and to novelty.

We have two rules for using this type of affirmation in action. It needs to be:

1. something that would delight the other person (not you),
2. random and unexpected.

One method for finding out what delights another person is to pay attention to "random droppings"—the little comments that people make about things they like and want—and to the treasures they hold close to their heart. A coworker who talked about how lilies remind her of her mother who has passed might be touched to find a bouquet of lilies on her desk one morning. A mom who framed your childhood note to Santa might cherish the new note you write, thanking her for making Christmas so magical in childhood. Not only does this unconditional gift deepen the connection between gifter and giftee, but it helps the gifter pay attention to the distinctions of the other as a separate being.

Write: What a Surprise!

Instructions: Pay attention to the random droppings and treasures from people in your life. Use the following chart to record these. Once a month, surprise someone from that list by giving them (with no expectations of return) the item.

 Tip: Create a Random Droppings List on your phone to record throughout the day.

RANDOM DROPPINGS AND TREASURES WORKSHEET

Who	What	When Gifted

Read: The Boomerang Effect of the Affirmation Process

The give-and-take of Affirmations:

- Increases trust and safety between people.
- Stimulates positive brain health:
  - ~ Triggers the hypothalamus, which releases dopamine, a feel-good neurochemical that plays an important role in many functions, including pleasure, reward, and motivation.
  - ~ Boosts serotonin production, the "happy chemical," as it contributes to feelings of well-being and helps us feel relaxed.
  - ~ Decreases cortisol, thereby lowering anxiety and relaxing defenses.
- Changes our worldview. Rather than living from a place of deficit, we will begin to experience a surplus of good.
- Ignites the boomerang effect. When we affirm unconditionally (no strings attached), it's as if we are giving it to ourselves.

Write: Flooding with Positives

Overview: Words matter. Actions matter. And the sum of words + actions is greater than the parts.

Through words and actions, the Positive Flooding Exercise invites the one-way sharing of positive affirmations with great energy and enthusiasm. The purpose of the Positive Flooding Exercise is to:

- amplify the positive energy in relationships,
- have intense emotion become associated with the positives rather than the negatives, and
- access and express life energy.

This process can be a challenge for both the speaker (to share positive things in a loud way) and the listener (who may not be used to hearing positive affirmations and/or equates loudness with anger). We recommend still doing the process but repeating it throughout the week to help overcome the resistance and create new neural pathways. While this might be a challenge for some, we guarantee that it is much better to flood in positivity than drown in negativity!

Instructions:

1. On the chart on the next page, list your practice partner's physical characteristics, personality traits, behaviors, and global affirmations that you appreciate, admire, and cherish. (Note: If you do not have a practice partner, invite a friend or family member to experience this powerful exercise. Explain the process ahead of time. Flood them first and invite—but don't require—them to flood you in return. Kids, by the way, love this, so consider flooding your child, nephew or niece, young cousin, etc.)

2. Decide who will be the first speaker. The listener sits in a chair in the middle of the room. The speaker slowly walks around the partner who is sitting, keeping eye contact whenever physically possible.

3. As the speaker, say all the wonderful things you wrote in your chart and others that come to mind. Flood your partner by beginning with your voice at its normal volume, then raise it a level after each category. Keep walking in a circle around the chair. Gradually speak louder and louder until you are shouting positive global expressions of care (for example, "You are the best friend ever!" or "I feel so lucky to have you in my life!").

4. Switch places and repeat the above process.

Positive Flooding			
Physical Characteristics	**Personality Traits**	**Behaviors**	**Global Affirmations**
Blue eyes	Funny	Call me back when I reach out to you.	Best friend I ever had!

Daily Do

- Continue Dialoguing with your practice partner using a conversation starter from page 37.
- Share an appreciation; once a week, share with someone new.
- Monitor your ZN using a calendar.
- Write in your Me-2-We Journal.
- Read out loud or meditate on each sentence of your relational vision.
- Practice the mirroring sentence stems every day and throughout the day.
- Practice emptying your mind by meditating, walking outside and focusing on your senses, and doing nothing (*niksen*).
- Be mindful of your assumptions about others.
- Practice curiosity ("Is there more about that?"or "I would love to hear more about that!").
- Pay attention to the random droppings and treasures that people hold (and add to your chart on page 113).

Monthly Do

- Surprise someone with a gift from your chart on page 116.
- Share a deep appreciation.
- Share a positive flooding once a month with someone new from your Easy bubble (page 8).

When you have completed the readings, Dialogue practice, and writing exercises, proceed to the next session.

Conflict Is Growth Trying to Happen

Review: Chapter 7

Introduction

When you are in a relationship with other people, there are three entities involved: you, them, and the Space-Between. That space can unite or separate the entities depending on whether it is filled with positive and productive energies or negative and polarizing energies. The spaces between you and your family, friends, coworkers, and other mortal beings include how we look at people, the tone of our voices, the body energies, our inner conscious and unconscious narratives, and, of course, our words.

Throughout this relational journey, you have explored this Space-Between by:

- creating a relational vision of how you see yourself in your relationships,
- committing to and practicing ZN,
- listening deeply and accurately by practicing the mirroring process and recognizing random droppings,
- replacing your need for certainty with not-knowing and curiosity,
- validating and discovering the other,
- deepening your empathy by discerning the roots under your triggers and frustrations and listening to others,

- translating frustrations into wishes,
- cultivating appreciations daily, and
- affirming others by intentionally implementing laughter, play, and unconditional gifts.

The more you practice these skills, the stronger your relational competency muscles will become. And the stronger the muscles, the greater your ability to hold your reactivity to provocations and foster meaningful connections.

In this session, you will continue thinking about your contribution to the polarization you might experience at times and grow into new behaviors by implementing SMART changes.

Read: My Way or the Highway!

When we hold a single point of view stubbornly and prevent another person from standing equally side by side, we risk greater rifts between "us" and "them." This dangerous refusal to acknowledge differences is the root cause of our diverging cultural, economic, ethnic, and political animosities. The assignments in this workbook have been designed to permit difference by peeling back to the layers underneath, embracing discomfort, and deploying the Wise Owl (higher brain) to communicate in a nonconfrontational way. But it is an ongoing process to:

- catch our prejudices and negative messages,
- explore our inner narratives,
- lessen our minimizing and maximizing tendencies, and
- broaden our perceptions through listening and curiosity.

Write: How Polarized Is My Thinking?

Instructions: Read the statements below and rate yourself on a scale of 1 to 5.

	Never (1)	Rarely (2)	Sometimes (3)	Often (4)	Always (5)
I immediately dismiss another's point of view because it's not my own.					
I make people feel guilty when they do not comply with my wishes.					
I interrupt other people when they say something I disagree with.					
I repeatedly point out what others are doing wrong.					
I refuse to listen to information that someone genuinely wishes to share.					
I assume other people know what I expect of them and are upset with them when they don't.					
I seldom ask for feedback but give feedback to others.					
I interrupt people before they finish expressing an opinion that differs from my own.					

Me-2-We Journey: When Do I Dehumanize?

The polarized mind often leads to a tendency to dehumanize. Dehumanizing someone or groups of people is fodder for war propaganda and for political votes. And it also, in subtler ways and on a smaller scale, influences who we befriend and who we push away, where we live, how we raise our children, where we work, and how we treat people in our everyday lives. Those we isolate from can become unworthy of our compassion or empathy and worthy of inhumane treatment, or even physical or emotional annihilation. The posts we like or share on social media, and the jokes we tell or laugh at, often perpetuate these prejudices in less-extreme forms.

Instructions: Think about times when you either used or thought dehumanizing terms (overt or subtle) to perpetuate a prejudice of a person or a group of people, such as using:

- animal or insect metaphors (beasts, vermin, animals, pigs, gorillas, leeches, etc.);
- synonyms with *evil* (satanic, devilish, unholy, vile, wicked, etc.);
- labels that stigmatize or categorize a person, such as an ex-convict or addict;
- nonhuman terms, such as *aliens*.

Spend five to ten minutes writing down your memories on the next page or in your Me-2-We Journal.

Tip: When You Don't See Eye to Eye

Sentence Stems to Share Your Perspective:

- "My perspective on this topic is . . ."
- "Would you be willing to share with me your perspective on this topic?"
- "From listening to you, a new perspective I got is . . ."
- "In my view, where we share common ground is . . ."
- "What I would like to better understand is . . ."

Dialogue: Frustration Dialogue

Purpose: Experiencing frustrations is universal. Using this Dialogue will keep you connected rather than polarized.

Instructions: Spend a few minutes reviewing your frustrations list on page 67. Choose a mild frustration (something that does not have a lot of energy attached to it), and share with your practice partner using the Frustration Dialogue.

Prompts for Speaker:

- "Is now a good time to share a recent frustration I had with someone?"
- "I was frustrated when . . ."
- "The story I make up about the person is . . ."
- "When I experienced that behavior, I felt . . ."
- "And I reacted by . . ."
- "That feeling reminds me of . . ."
- "What I long for or what I wish were different is . . ."

Prompts for Listener:

- Mirrors, checks for accuracy, and asks, "Is there more about that?"
- Asks deepening questions, such as:
    - ~ "What would you like to be different?"
    - ~ "What can I do to reduce your frustration about that?"
- When there is no more:
    - ~ summarize (and check for accuracy),
    - ~ validate (and check for accuracy),
    - ~ empathize (and check for accuracy).

Tips: Stop and Think

Are all frustrations about me or my past? No, not always. But a sure sign that a frustration is more about you than about the other depends on:

1. the intensity of the frustration (the greater the tension, the more likely there is an underlying narrative), and
2. whether it is repetitive. For example, if you use words like *always* ("You are always late") or *never* ("You never consider others!"), you are using telltale signs that there's a relational story underneath.

If at any point you are feeling very emotional about an interaction, try to move away from the experiential and into the cognitive by asking yourself questions, such as:

- What do I think is happening right now?
- Is this feeling familiar?
- Where do I think these feelings are from?
- What is my fear underneath?
- What is the story I tell myself?
- What is my wish under this feeling?

Read: Embrace the Wise (and SMART) Owl!

While we may not be able to control others, we can control our choices.

To become more relationally competent, you can create a behavioral change that stretches you to reach a relational goal. Behavioral change is an opportunity for growth and requires a positive and SMART gift to optimize success.

- **S**mall and specific (a behavior you can see)
- **M**easurable (an observer could count the number of times when it is happening)
- **A**ttainable (a small step)
- **R**elevant (to the statement)
- **T**ime-limited (for example, once a day for two weeks)

Write: SMART Gifts for Change

Instructions:

Review your relational vision on page 24 and choose an "easy" statement. Then write that statement in the space below (*easy* means something that you are relatively successful at already but could use some improvement).

In my relational vision, I _____

_____.

Based on that vision statement, answer the following:

The reason this is important to me is _____

_____.

On a scale of 1 (poor) to 5 (fabulous), where I see myself being now is _____.

One thing I could do this week to increase this number by half a point is _____

_____.

One way I might stop myself from doing this is _____

_____.

When I imagine doing this in my life all the time, I feel _____

_____.

Now, create and write in the appropriate space a SMART behavior you can integrate (with some stretching) to gift yourself on your relational journey.

Example:

In my relational vision, I am a good listener.

Behavior Change:

> Time Frame: When I go out with Jenn on Friday
>
> Specific Behavior Change: I will focus more on listening and asking her questions, mirroring, and discovering something new about her.
>
> Relational Vision: _____
>
> Time frame: _____ (e.g., "In the next week" or "This Saturday morning")
>
> Specific Behavior Change: I will _____
>
> (specific behavior change that involves stretching).

Next, translate this vision statement into a specific objective and strategy and complete the Implementing My Relational Vision Worksheet, imagining the sensations of this gift (page 134). A sample is on page 133.

 Tips:

- Each gift of change should involve a "stretch," a new behavior that requires moving out of your comfort zone.

- Remember: *small steps*. Start with changes that you know you can commit to.

- Be forgiving of yourself. If at first you don't succeed, try, try again and consider the why. Did something unexpected happen? Did you find too many excuses to put it off? Alter your SMART change to make it more realistic and doable.

- Create a support system to help you be accountable (such as your practice partner). You can use Dialogue to see what worked, what didn't work, what emotions you experienced were, and how you would like to revise the SMART change.

- Celebrate when you are successful! Treat yourself. Revisit and revise the behavior change to continue integrating toward your relational goal.

- Create a new calendar that monitors your daily success. Give yourself a happy face or a frowny face each day. This will help you be intentional on a daily basis to achieve your relational goal.

- Spend a few minutes daily imagining that you have integrated this behavior change and the sensations associated with this change.

Implementing My Relational Vision Worksheet Sample		
Vision	I am a good listener.	
Objectives	I listen to people to understand and learn more about them before I respond.	
Strategy or Tactic	Mirror. Be curious and ask questions. Learn something new about Jenn.	Time Frame: 2 weeks
Sensory Effect	Imagine what it feels like living this. Taste: Sweetness Touch: Softness Smell: Roses Sound: Quiet Feel: Connected Emotions Experienced: Relaxed and proud	

Implementing My Relational Vision Worksheet	
Vision	
Objectives	
Strategy or Tactic	Time Frame:
Sensory Effect	Imagine what it feels like living this. Taste: Touch: Smell: Sound: Feel: Emotions:

Dialogue: Gifts of Change

Instructions: With your practice partner, using the Gifts of Change Dialogue, share the SMART behavioral change you chose to activate in your relational vision.

Prompts for Speaker:

- "Is now a good time to share a gift of change?"
- "The relational vision statement I decided to work on is . . ."
- "My feelings and/or fears about that are . . ."
- Listen to the mirror, summary, validation, and empathy. Then respond to the listener's questions:
    - ~ "One thing I will do to help me grow and fulfill my relational vision is . . ."
    - ~ "When I do this, I imagine I will feel . . ."
- "Thank you for listening."

Prompts for Listener:

- Mirror, check for accuracy, and invite more throughout.
- When there is no more:
    - ~ summarize (and check for accuracy),
    - ~ validate (and check for accuracy),
    - ~ empathize (and check for accuracy).
- Then ask: "What would you like to do that would help you grow and fulfill your relational vision?" or "When you stretch into this change, how do you think you will feel?"
- "Thank you for sharing."

Daily Do

- Continue Dialoguing with your practicing partner.
- Share an appreciation.
- Monitor your ZN using a calendar.
- Write in your Me-2-We Journal.
- Read out loud or meditate on each sentence of your relational vision.
- Practice the mirroring sentence stems every day and throughout the day.
- Practice emptying your mind by meditating, walking outside and focusing on your senses, and doing nothing (*niksen*).
- Be mindful of your assumptions about others.
- Practice curiosity. Every time you feel reactive, get curious! Explore what this situation tells you about yourself. The aim is to bring the unconscious to the conscious.
- Pay attention to the random droppings and treasures that people hold (and add to your chart on page 113).
- Spend a few minutes imagining that you have integrated your SMART behavior change and the sensations associated with this change.

Monthly Do

- Share a deep appreciation with someone new.
- Continue reviewing your Challenging and Impossible relational bubbles (page 9) to discover more about yourself.
- Surprise someone with an unconditional gift from your chart on page 116.
- Share a positive flooding with someone new from your Easy bubble (page 8).
- Review your relational vision, edit as needed, and implement a new SMART behavior change.

Proceed to the next session once you have successfully engaged in a new behavior.

We Just Need a Little Brain Surgery

Review: Chapter 11

Introduction

Modern science continues to discover more about our amazing brain. One new discovery is that our brains have the ability to create new brain cells and neural connections throughout one's lifetime. Your brain can change its structure in response to new experiences, regardless of your age. This is called *neuroplasticity*. You *can* teach an old dog new tricks!

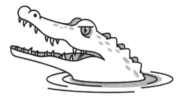

The SC process gives us the ability to harness the power of this neuroplasticity. By managing our thoughts, reactions, and behaviors, we employ our cognitive and rational abilities. Through practice, experience, and repetition, we strengthen our emotional regulation skills and increase our synaptic connections. Practicing the SC Dialogue rescues us from the Crocodile (lower brain) mode and invites us to think, feel, and operate from the Wise Owl (higher brain) mode. Instead of unfiltered words pouring out of our mouths, we learn to tolerate ambiguity, which is our ability to handle uncertainty, unpredictability, and conflict.

A sign of mental health is this capacity to stay with uncomfortable feelings, while allowing space for others to share their experience and perspective. The SC Dialogue provides a structure for holding this ambiguity when we are feeling reactive: we slow down, focus on the other, become curious, and move into our higher brain. Our conscious efforts override our instinctive reactions.

Human relationships are layers of narratives, made up of our lifelong experiences, interactions, and biology. These narratives contribute to our reactions.

In this session, we will explore additional ways to understand our reactivity so that we can strengthen our inner Wise Owl to keep the inner Crocodile from hijacking the relational space with an escalation of words.

Write: A Turtle and a Hailstorm Meet at a Bar

Overview: The primary function of the Crocodile Brain is to keep us alive and defend us from harm. If the lower brain perceives something as dangerous (real or imaginary), the alarm goes off, the neurochemicals (adrenaline and cortisol) start flowing, and the body goes on full alert and responds with a fight, flight, or freeze stance—an expansion or reduction of physical energy.

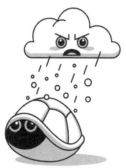

In our SC work, we call these adaptations *Turtles* (minimizers) and *Hailstorms* (maximizers). In response to perceived danger, Turtles tend to react by holding or toning down their energy: defending themselves by swallowing their emotions and/or retreating into their shells. Hailstorms, in contrast, tend to expand their internal energy outward: magnifying everything and/or making everything into a crisis. Because they affect how we relate to others, and in return, how others relate to us, it is important to identify the defensive strategy you typically use when you feel threatened.

Instructions: Study the descriptions on the next page, circle the items that you think best describe you when you feel threatened. Based on those answers, determine if you are a Turtle or a Hailstorm. Although all of us express both Turtle and Hailstorm responses, depending on the context, usually one is our main response, and we usually function in opposition to the people who have the other response.

How to Talk with Anyone about Anything Workbook

Am I a Turtle?

When I get upset, I tend to:

- Feel tight inside and do not verbalize my emotions.
- Adopt an "I'll take care of myself/I don't need anyone" attitude.
- Express very few, if any, needs and exclude others from my personal space.
- Listen poorly and attempt to figure things out by myself.
- Remove myself from my relationships without explanation.

Am I a Hailstorm?

When I get upset, I tend to:

- Express myself with passion and energy, using many words.
- Repeat myself and interrupt others to get their attention.
- Feel an intense need for a response and persist until I get one.
- Express many needs and listen poorly when others are talking.
- Adopt a victim stance and blame others for what I am experiencing.

Draw: Turtles Turtling and Hailstorms Hailing

The greater the hailstorm, the greater the turtle retreats!

Instructions: Doodle your best Turtle in a Hailstorm (and feel free to add labels).

Tips: When You Feel Upset, Try Singing!

While "music has charms to soothe the savage breast, to soften rocks, or bend a knotted oak,"[1] music's cousin—singing—may calm (at least) the Crocodile. Much research has touted the mental and physical health benefits of singing. Here are just a few pluses for belting it out:

- **Brain exercise:** When we speak, the hemisphere of the brain dealing with language lights up. When we sing, though, both hemispheres light up, including the area that controls emotions.[2] Singing also releases endorphins, the brain's feel-good chemicals. Given that singing utilizes different parts of the brain, we consider warbling to be a full neural workout!

- **Stress buster:** A 2015 study showed that the amount of stress hormone released is reduced after singing—whether people are singing in a group or by themselves.[3]

- **A sense of belonging and connection:** When you sing with others, you're likely to feel the same kind of camaraderie that players on a sports team experience. And when people feel bonded together, the neurochemical oxytocin (a.k.a. the love hormone) is released. Singing in a group can evoke a sense of community, well-being, and social inclusion.[4] So next time you are singing during the seventh-inning stretch or during church Mass, you are also increasing your sense of self-worth and belonging.

- **Physical workout:** Singing is an aerobic exercise that stimulates the immune response,[5] increases the pain threshold,[6] and improves lung function and circulation.[7] Sounds much more fun than an hour at the gym!

So the next time you are feeling stressed, try using your vocal cords to carry your favorite tune (but make sure you are singing in a place that won't make you anxious, as that might produce more cortisol![8]). Consider adding solo singing to your daily workout (such as in the shower or on your way to work) with songs from your favorite decade and embrace opportunities for group singing (such as in a faith choir group or with your chums at a local bar singing "The Irish Rover").

Me-2-We Journey: Opposites Attract

Did you know? Opposites *do* attract! Turtles and Hailstorms usually find each other and fall in love. Think about your past intimate relationships and/or your current intimate relationship and the times where there was tension in the relationship. Consider the following prompts:

- How did I react? What did I do? What did I say? What did I feel?
- How did my partner react? What did they do? What did they say? What did they feel?
- What could I have done differently?

Spend at least five minutes writing what comes to mind in the space below (or write in your Me-2-We Journal).

Dialogue: Turtle-Hailstorm Dialogue

Instructions: With your practice partner, use SC Dialogue to share how you react to tension.

Prompts for Speaker:

- "I would like to have a Dialogue about how I express my energy when I am upset. Is now a good time?"
- "First, I would like to express an appreciation to you, which is _____."
- "When I am upset, I tend to be like a _____ [Turtle or Hailstorm] and _____ [choose an item circled on page 142] to protect myself."
- "When I think about that, I feel_____."
- "When I get upset, what I experience in my body is _____."
- "When I feel reactive toward someone, the story I make up about them is _____."
- "And when I feel that, it reminds me that when I was little and felt threatened, I _____."

Note: If you are not comfortable sharing something from your childhood with your practice partner, you can opt to share a memory of how you reacted in a past intimate relationship.

Prompts for Listener:

- Mirror, check for accuracy, and invite more throughout.
- When there is no more:
    - ~ summarize (and check for accuracy),
    - ~ validate (and check for accuracy), and
    - ~ empathize (and check for accuracy).

Tips: Taming the Hailstorm and Inviting the Turtle Out of Its Shell

Now that you have identified how you react when you feel upset or threatened, it's time to employ the Wise Owl to engage in new behaviors and rewrite your script. While you may not be able to control your first feeling or thought of discomfort, you can control your second. We call this the *stretching principle*, which is the act of going beyond your comfort zone into new territory.

Hailstorm Tips:

- Hijack your energy into something else. Knit. Take a walk. Call a friend. Read. Breathe deeply. Sing!
- When you feel calmer, ask for a Dialogue and use "I" language, focusing on how *you* are feeling. Make sure you use succinct messages so you don't overwhelm the Turtle and cause them to retreat back into their shell.

Turtle Tips:

- Mirror, mirror, mirror. Hailstorms often just need to be heard and seen.
- Honor your need for space by saying, "I need some time for myself to process. Can we have a SC Dialogue to discuss this in an hour?" And then initiate the Dialogue. Make sure you use "I" messages and focus on how *you* feel (and share the layers underneath the feeling).

Read: What Does This Say About Me?

Projection is a psychological term that describes a defense mechanism: we unconsciously assign to someone else something about ourselves that is undesirable, such as a trait or a feeling.

We project all the time. Sometimes these projections are something that we already know about ourselves. Sometimes it triggers a suppressed memory about a bad experience. Sometimes it's something in ourselves that we refuse to accept. Here's an example.

Once upon a time, I (Harville) shared an office with a psychiatrist friend named James, and we decided to find a third office mate. James had a friend who was interested. A few days later, I saw a man walking down the hall away from me. And there was something about his walk that irritated me. I immediately thought to myself, *What an arrogant man!* Once I met this person, whose name was Robert, I found him very pleasant with not a hint of arrogance, and eventually we became good friends. What happened? I had projected my own arrogance onto Robert.

It's easier to see when someone projects onto you. ("Well, ain't that the pot calling the kettle black!") It's a lot more difficult to notice when you're the one projecting. Here are some signs that you might be projecting:

- feeling overly defensive or sensitive about something someone has said or done
- feeling highly reactive and quick to blame
- making an assumption about someone

So when we find an irritating trait about another, it's an opportunity to explore what that means about ourselves.

Me-2-We Journey: I Am ~~Nothing~~ Something Like Them

Refer back to the following:

- the three negative traits you circled on the My Relational Profile chart (page 10)
- the three people you circled on the relational Challenging and Impossible bubbles (page 9).

Think about the following:

- Are any of the traits I find intolerable also in myself?
- How have I, in the past, possessed one of these traits? What did I do?
- In what ways have I been like this person?
- Who or what does this person remind me of?

Using one of the following prompts, spend at least five minutes writing what comes to mind in the space on the next page (or write in your Me-2-We Journal).

- I am like _____ [person from Challenging or Impossible bubble] in the following ways . . .
- I am _____ [negative trait] in the following ways . . .

Bonus: Share this information with your practice partner using Dialogue.

Write: Do You Resist Gifts?

Overview: Do you know that we can fear pleasure? Think of a time when you were uncomfortable receiving a gift and pushed it back. Or a time when you received a compliment but then turned the compliment around to compliment the other person. Were you uncomfortable being flooded with positives in session 5? Do you recognize yourself in any of the statements below?

- I am uncomfortable when someone brags about me.
- When I receive a gift, I feel obligated to reciprocate somehow.
- I have refused gifts, saying they were unnecessary.
- I deflect compliments when I get them.
- I feel uncomfortable wanting things for myself.
- I feel uncomfortable asking for what I want or need.

Many of us struggle with receiving. Often our inability to receive gifts stems from the messages we received in childhood such as, "You are not worthy enough," "You should have fewer needs," or "Beware! Gifts come with a price tag."

Instructions: Think about times you received a gift that you deflected or rejected. It could have been a compliment or a physical gift. Using the chart on the next page, write down the gift, who gave it, and your memory of your feeling when you received the gift.

Going forward, continue recording the gifts you have trouble receiving. Explore why you might feel you don't deserve this, what it reminds you of, and what assumptions you have of the gift. And practice stretching when you receive the gift by:

- saying "Thank you" and not deflecting,
- letting go of any assumptions that the gift is conditional, and
- telling yourself, "I deserve this."

Receiving Inventory			
When	What	Who	I felt ...

Daily Do

- Continue Dialoguing with your practice partner, using a conversation starter from page 37.
- Share an appreciation. Once a week, share with someone new.
- Monitor your ZN using a calendar.
- Write in your Me-2-We Journal.
- Read out loud or meditate on each sentence of your relational vision.
- Practice the mirroring sentence stems every day and throughout the day.
- Practice emptying your mind by meditating, walking outside and focusing on your senses, and doing nothing (*niksen*).
- Be mindful of your assumptions about others.
- Practice curiosity. Every time you feel reactive, get curious! Explore what this situation tells you about yourself. The aim is to bring the unconscious to the conscious.
- Pay attention to the random droppings and treasures that people hold (and add to your chart on page 113).
- Spend a few minutes imagining that you have integrated your SMART behavior change and the sensations associated with this change.
- Monitor your inability to receive and continue recording moments on the chart on page 153.
- Consider adding singing to your daily routine.

Monthly Do

- Surprise someone from your chart on page 116.
- Share a deep appreciation.
- Share a positive flooding with someone new from your Easy bubble (page 8).
- Continue reviewing your Challenging and Impossible relational bubbles (page 9) to discover more about yourself.
- Review your relational vision, edit as needed, and implement a new SMART behavior change.

Proceed to the next session once you feel that (1) you have become more conscious of how you react during tension and conflict, and (2) your Wise Owl muscles are strengthening.

Relational Competency in Every Aspect of Life

Review: Chapters 8–10 and 12

Introduction

SC tools create a level playing field in conversations, where any topic can be calmly discussed regardless of age, gender, or roles. When we move away from our pain and blame, we bring an appreciation for our world so that safety and joy can be restored within our families and communities. It can be gentle yet fierce work as we become proponents and advocates of relationships and equality. It is soulful, heartful, and meaningful.

In these pages, you have practiced the four skills to obtain and strengthen your relational competency:

1. A structured Dialogue
2. Empathy with everyone
3. The ZN commitment
4. The practice of Affirmations

These skills can be applied everywhere, all the time, and with everyone—from civic organizations, service industries, political forums, corporations, and religious communities to more personal relationships, such as family, intimate relationships, friends and colleagues, and, of course, in our everyday interactions. Not only do these skills foster connection and increase collaboration, but they also are tools to de-escalate tension or conflict and establish a safe space to honor differences. Remember: we all want to be heard, seen, and valued. And to accomplish that goal, we need to hear, see, and value others.

In this last session, we will explore ideas to apply these four relational competency skills to different ecosystems—*living, working, learning,* and *worshiping.* And while they are suggestions, the applications are endless. The first item we will review is Group Dialogue.

Read: SC Group Dialogue (Communologue)

Group Dialogue is a guided conversation that creates a safe space in which members of a group can discuss, share, and process information or support, reconnect, explore, preempt conflict, and/or facilitate community building. Similar to a SC Dialogue between two people, Group Dialogue is an open-ended process without an inherent outcome or result (Group Reflection), but it can, if the group chooses, prepare the ground for the group to reach a simple agreement or make a decision through consensus (Group Solution). It can also equip decision-makers to choose a direction that reflects the "mind" of the group.

Group Dialogue Guidelines:

1. ZN is the agreed-upon norm.
2. Everyone is invited to speak but is not required to do so.
3. Cross talk is avoided (because it creates a dyad instead of community sharing).
4. Every viewpoint is regarded as valid.
5. Expressions of diversity are encouraged, while debate is discouraged.
6. Statements that imply absolutes and objective "truth" are avoided.
7. Sharing is brief and clear.
8. Mirroring is directed to the center of the group and in third person, such as "What I heard Bob say was . . ." This reduces reactivity by providing distancing.
9. Members commit to confidentiality. What happens in a Group Dialogue stays in the Group Dialogue.

GROUP LEADER ROLE:

A group leader is identified. Their role is to:

1. Ensure the agenda, objective, time allotted, and people involved are determined prior to the Group Dialogue.
2. Establish the structure of the Dialogue. There are two types of sharing:
   a. Sequential: In a particular order (such as starting from the left of the group leader and moving around a circle clockwise). However, group members are not required to share and are given the option to skip their turn.
   b. Random or Popcorn sharing: There is no order. People can raise their hands when they have something to share and wait for the group leader to call on them.
3. Guide members to adhere to the Group Dialogue guidelines. For example, if an absolute is stated, the group leader can ask the member to resend the sharing in a different way or can do a mirroring intervention to restore a sharing tone. Examples:

   Speaker: This is a fact.
   Leader: If I hear that, Julie believes . . .
   Speaker: This is what happened.
   Leader: Randall's perspective on what happened is that . . .

4. Monitor sharing time. Sharing time should be determined at the start of the meeting (such as one or two minutes per person). If one member seems to be dominating the sharing, then gently level the field by giving a short mirror, thanking them, and asking, "Let's hear from someone else."
5. Determine roles for mirroring and summarizing. This can be completed by the group leader or randomly (e.g., "Who would like to mirror Joe?").
6. Remain neutral at all times. This is essential to maintain the safety of the group. The priority of the group leader is the process, not the content.

GROUP DIALOGUE STEPS:

1. Group leader identifies the intention and announces the agenda. This can be done at the beginning of the meeting or announced prior to the gathering.

2. Group leader begins the meeting by inviting appreciations (to either the group as a whole or from any member sharing publicly an appreciation of another member).

3. Group leader invites discussion on the topic.

4. Group members share within the fixed time frame.

5. Speakers are mirrored by another group member:

   a. "If I got it, _____ [name of speaker] said _____. Did I get it?"

   b. Once the speaker is mirrored by the listener, other group members may volunteer to mirror something they may have heard that the original listener had missed. "I also heard _____ [name of speaker] share _____. Did I get that as well?"

 6. When the sharing is complete, one member of the group offers a summary that captures the main points.

7. If time permits, group members can briefly share their experience with the process. Offering a sentence stem will facilitate this process, such as, "This process has made me feel . . ." or "What I learned today was . . ."

If the goal is for consensus on some actionable item, then after the consensus develops through summary or continued sharing:

1. a plan of action evolves,

2. a timeline is created,

3. tasks are identified and assigned, and

4. the group reconvenes at another time that is determined at the end of the meeting.

 TIPS AND OPTIONS:

- Depending on the group size and time, the Group Dialogue can move into smaller working groups, using the same guidelines, and then come back together as a large group to share the main takeaways.

- While not necessary in group settings, a group member or leader can validate and empathize with the speaker, especially if the sharing is emotion-laden.

Living: Safe Conversations in Our Homes

For many of us, the most contentious relationships begin at home. And yet, most of us want our family relationships to work. That's why SC Dialogue can be the most useful household tool ever created. Here are some ideas of specific applications to the family unit.

DIALOGUE:

- **Couples:** Our work with couples was launched with our book *Getting the Love You Want*. Our three-step Dialogue has helped millions of couples not only save their marriage from divorce but also develop a thriving relationship. They probably benefit the most from Dialogue due to the tension that develops only in an intimate dyad because of the unique nature of romantic attraction. And what better gift to give your children than to provide them with a model for a healthy and happy marriage? We strongly encourage couples to make a commitment to use the Dialogue skills with each other to protect and nourish their relationship.
- **Parent-Child:** Parents who mirror, validate, and empathize with their children (or their coparent) are modeling commitment to the practice of everyone's being heard, seen, and valued.

Imago therapist and SC Leader Morella Hammer has found Dialogue extremely valuable for the Hispanic families with whom she works. It bridges the gap between immigrant parents and their first-generation American children, along with the tension between cultural identity and tradition when blending in and adopting an American attitude.

A lot of the first-generation kids felt they did not have a voice, as their parents came from a cultural system embedded in a "follow my rules" dictate. Dialogue helped the kids find a voice and feel safe enough to have those hard conversations with their parents about school issues and family expectations.[1]

Here's another story shared by an Imago therapist, Dawn Lipthrott, about one of her clients:

Mary had two boys, nine and seven years old. One day the older boy took one of the younger brother's toys and they started fighting and crying. Mary went into the living room and asked what happened. She mirrored just the main points, asked if there was more—and there was. She continued mirroring the basic points, told the other one when he interrupted that she would listen to him, too, in just a minute, and then expressed understanding about why it made perfect sense that the one talking was upset. The boy was nodding as she expressed understanding. And then she did the same for the brother.

About a week later, one of the boys came home upset about something that happened at school and said, "Can we talk like that weird way we did about the toy?" Mary couldn't believe it, and did.[2]

You are never too young, or too old, to experience the power of being heard.

When his children were young, Imago faculty member and friend Dr. Wade Luquet would take them on WOW Walks. Their mission was to discover any amazing nuance in nature, which they would point to and yell, "Wow!" and explain to the others the "why in the wow." Then the others would mirror the "Wow!" and add any additional observations. Through this connecting family experience, the boys became more aware of their surroundings, practiced mirroring in a unique way, and expressed joy through inflated voices.

GROUP DIALOGUE:

We recommend Group Dialogues to learn the basic tools of Dialogue and value everyone's voice in the family. Here are some ideas:

- Create a Family Circle hour.
- Implement it regularly (such as every Sunday morning) rather than "as needed." It's important to view the Family Circle time as a fun and safe space rather than a warning that "there's a problem."
- Use Group Dialogues to brainstorm family vacation ideas, household expectations, weekend activities, or to come up with a sentence stem for everyone to share, such as "One thing that happened at school/work this week that made me happy is . . ."
- When frustrations are expressed, help kids find the wish that is disguised in the frustration.

- Teach the Dialogue skills and have all members practice Dialogue using speaker and listener responsibility (for younger kids, mirroring is a great start).
- End the Family Circle time with high-energy, such as dancing around, jumping up and down while trying to recite a tongue twister, or having a contest on the most exaggerated and funniest laugh.

AFFIRMATIONS:

- Start family meetings by reading the 7 A's (page 104) and change the "I" to "We."
- Practice Affirmation Dialogues in the family unit (page 110).
- Have family members work together to plan surprises for another family member.
- Create an appreciation jar for each family member. Have family members intentionally capture appreciations on pieces of paper. Jars can be opened and read on special occasions, such as a birthday, or when a pick-me-up is needed. Be creative—have an art box nearby filled with colorful pieces of paper, magazines, a pair of scissors, crayons, watercolors, and paintbrushes.
- Institute a family appreciation ritual that occurs regularly, such as every night at the dinner table.
- Be giving with your appreciations, including having your child/children witness appreciations to your spouse, friends, and other family members.
- Positive Flooding: Kids love not only being a recipient but also flooding other family members! You can do this regularly (but no more than once a month), alternating family members, use on special occasions, or employ when a particular family member needs a pick-me-up. Family members can even request a flooding (teaching them that it is okay to ask for what you need!).

ZERO NEGATIVITY:

Not only have we practiced Dialogue in our own family, but we also instituted a Family Protocol (see the next page). The protocol adheres to the ZN principles, of which we regularly remind our children if there is a breakdown. Be sure to discuss signals for put-downs, which can be during Family Circle time.

Harville and Helen's Family Protocol

Hello, family!

We have a commitment to ZN. It suggests all conversations be expressed kindly.

If you ever feel hurt by someone, say "Marshmallow," "Ouch," or "Bing." This means, "Can you say that in another way that doesn't feel negative to me?"

Do not be negative back.

Suggested guidelines while we are all together:

1. If you become frustrated with anyone, ask them for an appointment and request a Dialogue.
2. Express any frustration kindly, using Speaker Responsibility so that the other person can "hear" you.
3. The person listening should use the three steps of Dialogue (mirroring, validating, and empathizing).
4. The person listening can then kindly accept what the other person has said or may ask for a Dialogue with the other person to express their own view.
5. Remember: validating does not mean that you agree with what the other person has said but that you care and respect that person and their point of view.

It is a moment of triumph when you repair and restore connection! It's time to celebrate!

Don't forget, mistakes are going to happen. People are going to get triggered. The sign of a great relationship is a quick repair.

Working: Safe Conversations in the Workplace

We believe the practice of SC Dialogue helps employees reach their full potential and, by extension, companies will see improvements to their bottom line. Employees and managers with strong interpersonal skills will lead the way to a healthier, more collaborative work environment. Engaged employees lead to less absenteeism and increased motivation and innovation and a greater ability to collaborate, be creative, problem solve, and think critically. While it is beneficial to have official SC training—especially in the management and human resources departments—it is absolutely possible to teach these basic skills and have everyone integrate them into their lives. SC Dialogue is useful for:

- HR issues
- colleague-to-colleague communications
- employer-to-employee relations
- customer service interactions (mirroring, validating, and empathizing with customers)

Role-playing various scenarios is helpful for all employees to teach and practice the skill.

GROUP DIALOGUE:

Businesses can use Group Dialogue for community building, creative brainstorming, and decision-making. Training through role-playing is especially beneficial (specifically in customer service interactions). Group Dialogue is also useful for board meetings, team meetings, and virtual meetings. (For virtual meetings, the group leader identifies two people ahead of time—"First Joe, then Mary"—and continues until everyone on the call has shared.) Group Dialogue meetings can focus purely on a conversation starter, such as:

- "A reason why a customer might go to our competitor is . . ."
- "What makes a great employee is . . ."
- "What makes an inspiring manager is . . ."
- "An idea on how to build rapport among the team is . . ."
- "A way to save money in the company is . . ."

Have team members become a part of the solution and share the collective wisdom through-out the company ranks.

AFFIRMATIONS:

- Appreciations:
  - ~ Sharing circle: Have everyone share one thing about the group or a particular person.
  - ~ Popcorn style: Start every meeting with a time for anyone to express an appreciation about anyone else. They can raise their hand, stand up, and so on, and say, "I have an appreciation for _____ [person's name]" and that person can mirror back the appreciation and express gratitude.
- Recognize an employee of the day/week/month: The group offers accolades about the chosen individual during a meeting or special occasion. This floods one person at a time, which can be impactful for both the recipient and the participants.
- Incorporate team play: Pajama Fridays, No Shave Novembers, Family BBQs, or team-building events, such as Karaoke Friday Fiesta. Assign a Team Play Committee and have members alternate once a quarter.
- Start business meetings with breaking into a dyad for the first five minutes and have every person share a quick appreciation about the other person (and mirror the response):
  - ~ "I appreciate that you are super responsive to emails!"
  - ~ "I appreciate how you break out in dance in front of the water cooler!"
  - ~ "I appreciated it when you helped me last Friday with the deadline."

ZERO NEGATIVITY:

- Create a "Zero Negativity Zone" sign at the work entrance that says, "Leave all criticism, shame, and blame behind!"
- Implement an HR policy that incorporates Dialogue for conflict resolution and a request for repair when connection has been ruptured.

The goal is to create a relational culture at work. It might feel artificial and rigid at first, but the flow comes with practice.

Here are some examples of people using the SC tools in the business environment:

SC Leader Nancy Bryant is a financial advisor who often has couples come to her office to create a retirement plan. She helps them identify their retirement vision ("What would retirement look like for you?") and begins with the partner who has the least amount of control over the finances. By giving them a voice—often for the first time—about money, Nancy often hears from the other partner something like, "I had no idea they had these ideas." Nancy then sends the couple away to talk—and listen—about their respective goals and find common ground. They then come back into her office to create a plan together based on their mutual vision. Dialogue helps them level the playing field by giving equal voice to their retirement vision.

Imago therapist Helit Assa took the tools unexpectedly to a work environment when she was having her hair done. She incorporated ZN, appreciations, request for change, and used Dialogue as the container to make that all happen. She recreated the scenario from memory:

I was at my salon appointment one time. Ben, my hairdresser, and his assistant, Rivka, were fighting about a client, and their voices were escalating throughout my time there. Toward the end of my haircut, I said to them, "Okay, let's talk about this in a healthy way." I asked them if they would be willing to go outside for a bit to work it through. They agreed.

We sat at a park bench just outside the salon. I looked at Ben and said, "Rivka has been an assistant with you for a very long time. Before we start, can you share something that you appreciate about her? Start with this sentence stem, 'I appreciate it when you . . . '"

He was embarrassed. "Well, she knows what I think about her."

"No, she doesn't. Say one thing. Look at her eyes when you say it."

After a while, he finally was able to say something simple like, "You do good work. I love how you work."

I asked Rivka to mirror the appreciation back to Ben. This made her uncomfortable but she was able to do it.

Then I turned to Rivka and said, "Can you share an appreciation you have for Ben?" She responded, "I love to work with you. You are very professional, and I learn from you."

Although uncomfortable because it was not "normal" for them, the shared appreciations cleared their heads from the argument.

I said to them, "I heard both of you inside the salon say, in different ways, that whatever you do, this client won't be satisfied. Is that accurate?"

They both confirmed that. "Yes. It's true."

"So why are you both fighting about her?"

Once they were able to see that they both agreed about the client, I asked them to tell each other how they felt about the situation and what they need from each other the next time. This is a variation of turning a frustration (which is a wish in disguise) into a specific request.

Rivka: I feel that you don't trust me in how I handle challenging clients. And I feel that you don't have my back—even behind the scenes and even when we know how difficult the client is.

(I guided Ben to mirror Rivka, check for accuracy, and ask for more, which took a few tries.)

Ben: So if I got it, you feel that I don't trust you and don't have your back when you are dealing with challenging clients. Did I get that? Is there more about that?

(After Rivka felt heard and there was no more, I guided Ben to turn the frustration into a request. This again took a few tries.)

Ben: What do you need for me to do differently so you feel respected and trusted by me?

Rivka: In the future, what would be helpful is when I am managing a difficult situation, you either (1) trust me fully in that process, or (2) pull me aside privately to discuss.

(The requests were then mirrored by Ben, and you could see the lightbulb go off when, on his own and without prodding, he said, "That makes sense. I can do that!" They both thanked each other and gave each other a high five with big grins on their faces.)

Then it was Ben's turn to share how he felt, the wish under his frustration, and the behavior-change request for the future. Similarly, Ben also felt an element of disrespect, describing how it played out when Rivka was yelling at him in front of other clients in the salon. After a bit of prodding, Ben requested that when a client called with a complaint, that Rivka would listen to the complaint and then let them know she will get back to them as soon as possible so she could process—either with him or on her own—rather than reacting to the client. And, similar to Rivka's request, he asked her to discuss in private if there was a need to discuss.

Both Ben and Rivka had similar frustrations, similar outlooks on this client, but because they were not listening to each other, their frustration played out in a reactive and defensive way, in front of a salon full of wide-eyed spectators.[3]

And that is "Safe Conversations at Work" in action!

Learning: Safe Conversations at Schools

As we have seen, it's never too early to start teaching and learning SC skills. Young students are quick to adapt and learn and practice. Here are some ideas for formally integrating the SC tools into schools.

SC DIALOGUE:

- Model in the classroom frequently.
  - ~ Teachers mirror students' questions.
  - ~ Students mirror questions and assignments.
- Students can be taught basic skills to navigate conflicts (by teachers, counselors, or administrative staff).
- Younger students can be shown how to navigate conflicts with teachers by taking on the mirroring role (as illustrated in Chapter 8 of the book, with the kindergarten class).
- Administrative staff can use Dialogue when advising students or handling disciplinary actions.
- Teachers can use Dialogue with parents on parent-teacher days and/or challenging parent conferences.
- School staff can handle interpersonal conflict between colleagues.
- Counselors can use Dialogue to bridge communication between parents and students.

GROUP DIALOGUE:

Schools can use Group Dialogue for staff meetings, school board meetings, student organizations, interactions between administration and students, and for any public group setting that invites an interactive process.

SC CONCEPTS:

In addition to teaching Dialogue skills, teachers can create lessons on other concepts and tailor them to the age group. Concepts can include:

- Introduction on the Brain
  - ~ Assign students to write (or illustrate) a story about a turtle caught in a hailstorm.

~ Give students a simple introduction to the brain and survival responses.

~ Tell a story about Wise Owl meeting the Cranky Crocodile (younger students can make puppets).

- "I" vs. "you" messages (and a worksheet on converting "you" messages into "I" messages)

- Students can role-play (using mirroring and Speaker Responsibility) different scenarios such as:

~ "Juan said I could not play soccer with them. That is so mean!"

~ "Hey, I was playing with that toy, and he took it! That is not fair!"

~ "Mom, you said we were going to the park today, and now we're not going."

AFFIRMATIONS:

- Celebrate a student (weekly, bimonthly, or monthly depending on the number of students in the classroom).

~ Have fellow classmates write on a piece of paper one thing they appreciate about the person.

~ Flood the student of the week by all students walking in a circle around the seated student, saying positive things about their physical characteristics, personality traits, and behaviors. At the end, everyone can jump up and down, shouting something like, "You are amazing!" or "You are so cool!"

- Have a Group Dialogue about what feels good (feathers) and what feels bad/sad (stones) and how buckets filled with feathers are light, but buckets filled with stones are heavy and are a burden to carry. Share ideas of how to fill buckets with feathers (be creative, such as "What fills your mom's bucket?" or "What fills your pet's bucket?").

ZERO NEGATIVITY:

Implement a ZN Zone in the classroom. Use Group Dialogue to (1) decide on a term for when someone experiences a put-down, and (2) determine options for repair. These should be visible in the classroom.

Worship: Safe Conversations in Religious Communities

Regardless of your religious and spiritual practice, the same ideas can be similarly applied to your community using Dialogue and Group Dialogue. Here are some stories of what this looked like for others:

- David Rudnick, who was board president of the Congregation Rodef Sholom in San Rafael, California, would start his monthly board meetings with an icebreaker question, such as "What is your favorite book?" Toward the end of his term, the board was meeting outside because of COVID-19. And instead of going around in their usual way (which was twenty-five people around a big table), David asked people to pair up. "I guided them to tell something about themselves and have the partner mirror it. My idea was that instead of the whole group learning about every single person, that using the technique of mirroring would create a deeper connection between two people. A quality of a functioning board is that people have strong connections with each other." Rabbi Elana Rosen-Brown recalled that meeting and shared: "I was paired up with David, and we found common ground when we discovered we both had parents who held on to our childhood homes. I remember looking around and seeing the deep resonance between people and that they could spend the entire evening talking. I also remember people asking, 'Can we do more of this?!'"[4]
- Religious communities offer wonderful resources to support families and marriages. Hold relationship workshops for members of your congregation: David, Rabbi Elana, Charlotte Legg, Harville, and Helen developed a workshop for relationship building around the High Holy Days and included a Dialogue around forgiveness. It was a powerful experience between couples. Here are some excerpts from a forgiveness Dialogue David had with his wife, Julie:
    - **Asking for an Appointment:** "Is now a good time to have a Dialogue so that I can share with you a behavior for which I would like to ask your forgiveness?"
    - **Sharing an Appreciation:** "One thing I appreciate about you is how you create opportunities for fun for our family even when we are feeling tired or weighed down by the world. Like going to the beach yesterday with Noah."
    - **Requesting Forgiveness:** "In the spirit of Teshuvah, I would like to ask now for forgiveness for sometimes being self-absorbed."

~ **Deepening:** "I can imagine that when I was oblivious and self-absorbed in this that you might have felt invisible, unappreciated, and unvalued. Is that what you thought or felt? Or do you have other thoughts or feelings that you would like to share?"

~ **Expressing a SMART Gift to the relationship.** "In the future, instead of being self-absorbed or self-focused, I will gift our relationship with three appreciations for you before every Shabbat for the next year to help enrich and make our relationship even better."

~ **Closings:** "Blessed is God, who gives us the ability to change, and commands us to seek forgiveness and perform Teshuvah as we enter a new year, so that we may return to our souls' essence." (*Hug*)

• Baldwin and Pollyanna Barnes directed family ministries at the Northeastern Conference of Seventh-Day Adventists. In September 2019, they were invited to Kenyatta University in Nairobi, Kenya, to participate in a ten-day program teaching the SC tools and methodology. As part of the program, they held two-hour sessions focusing on relational competencies. After each session, students were told to go into their community to practice what they learned, and they would come back the next day to share their experiences. Students reported back how the simplest three-word question, "Is there more?" helped them be more engaged with people, especially for students who were challenged with one-on-one conversations. In some cases, students brought their friends to the next session, who became curious about this new way to talk.

Often religious communities conduct formal ceremonies for certain rites of passage or milestones (such as birth, confirmation, bat/bar mitzvah, marriage, etc.) but can fall short on providing general ongoing support for relationship building. Relationship Gathering Groups can be a way for religious communities to develop stronger relationships among their members. Keep the conversations and purpose simple (it's not counseling). And remember, it's not the *what* of conversation but the *how* of conversation that fosters connection. Regular gatherings can:

~ utilize Group Dialogue to foster conversations,

~ guide members into sharing dyads,

~ teach concepts such as the Space-Between, and

~ share appreciations and challenges in a safe context.

Daily Do

- Dialogue, Dialogue, Dialogue. Be mindful of how you communicate (Speaker Responsibility) and strive to hear and understand others (Listener Responsibility).
- Share an appreciation—new, old, simple, deep. Mix it up on a daily basis!
- Regularly practice ZN in your thoughts, words, and actions. Even if your intentions are not negative, they might land negatively on others.
- Write in your Me-2-We Journal whatever comes to mind about your daily thoughts and experiences.
- Read or meditate on your relational vision, edit as needed, and continue to implement SMART behavior changes.
- Practice emptying your mind and strive for internal calmness.
- Be mindful of your assumptions about others. Rather than assume, practice curiosity!
- Pay attention to the random droppings and treasures that people hold.
- Whenever a relationship becomes challenging, pause and reflect on what this might mean about yourself.

Monthly Do

- Surprise someone with an unconditional gift.
- Share a positive flooding with someone.

Conclusion

Congratulations! You've made it! Think about how these past weeks have impacted your relational journey. How do you feel? What have you learned about yourself? What have you discovered about others? How have you grown?

When we give up the need to disprove the other and step into being present for them, relationships are transformed into a flow in which energy and information effortlessly oscillate. This resonance is singing together the music of connecting without judgment and experiencing a rhythm that is reliable and generative.

There is no end to this journey. These are lifetime skills with ever-evolving learnings. There is always more to know, discover, and understand. But, with practice, it gets easier. Armed with the tools of SC, *you* can be part of a global transformation by applying them to every facet of your life. We invite you to become a part of the solution, contributing toward a world where SC Dialogue is the new human language, and where we can live safely and joyfully together in community.

As a final step to celebrate your relational competency, let's revisit how you began this journey when you started this work with the RC Index.

Test Your Relational Competency

Instructions: Read each relational competency, description, and illustration and rate yourself from 1 to 10, with 10 as the highest score (i.e., I achieve that 100 percent of the time). When completed, compare with your score on page 17.

RELATIONAL COMPETENCY	DESCRIPTION	ILLUSTRATION	RATING (1-10)
Honoring boundaries	When I want to talk with someone, I check out in a warm voice tone whether they are available to listen at that time.	"Is now a good time to talk?"	
Honoring boundaries	When I want to talk and the person is not available at that time, I gently ask them to tell me when they are available and to let me know when that time comes.	"When would be a good time? And would you please come find me when the time comes?"	
Honoring boundaries	When someone wants to talk to me and I am not available at that time, I gently say when I can be available, and I initiate the conversation at the time I give them.	"I am not available right now, but I will be available in [minutes, hours, days]."	
Honoring boundaries	When I am available, in a warm tone of voice I let them know I am available.	"I am available now."	
Relaxing defenses	Before I start talking or listening, I make eye contact and take three deep breaths to relax my eyes and express my intention.	(*Makes eye contact, takes three breaths, and shares intention.*) "My intention is to stay connected to you while I am talking." "My intention is to stay connected to you while I am listening."	

RELATIONAL COMPETENCY	DESCRIPTION	ILLUSTRATION	RATING (1–10)
Expressing appreciations	When someone is available to listen to me, I express an appreciation for their availability.	"Thank you for being available to listen to what I want to say."	
Expressing appreciations	When someone says they are available to listen, I share an appreciation I have about them before I start talking.	"I have an appreciation for you that I want to share. When I see you do _____ [or hear you say _____], I really appreciate that."	
Speaker responsibility	When I speak with anyone, I start all my sentences with "I" rather than "you."	"Recently, I have been feeling _____, and I am curious about what you are thinking."	
Speaker responsibility	When I am talking, I describe my thoughts and feelings rather than describing the person who is listening.	"Sometimes I think _____, and when I think that I feel _____."	
Listener responsibility	When someone is talking to me and I get distracted or on overload, and can't listen anymore, I raise my hand and ask them to pause so I can mirror back what I heard so far, and then ask them to continue.	(Raises hand and says) "I would like to mirror what I have heard so far. If I got it, you said _____."	
Mirroring	After the person who is talking finishes their first few sentences, I mirror what I heard.	"Let me see if I am getting that. If I did, you said _____."	

RELATIONAL COMPETENCY	DESCRIPTION	ILLUSTRATION	RATING (1-10)
Checking for accuracy	After I mirror what I heard the other person say, I check with them to see if I got it accurately.	"Did I get that?" or "Did I get you accurately?"	
Checking for accuracy	When I summarize what I heard, I check with the speaker whether my summary is accurate.	"Did I get everything you said?"	
Checking for accuracy	After I share the feelings I see or imagine, I check to see if I got their feelings accurately.	"Is that the feeling?"	
Expressing curiosity	If they indicate I missed something, I ask them to send again the part I missed.	"Would you send again the part I missed?"	
Expressing curiosity	When the person I am listening to pauses, I ask them if they have more to say on the topic.	"Is there more about that?"	
Expressing curiosity	If the speaker says I did not get the feeling right, I ask them to share it again.	"Would you share your feeling with me again?"	
Expressing curiosity	After the feeling has been shared and confirmed, I ask if they have other feelings about that.	"Do you have other feelings about that?"	
Summarizing	When someone has finished speaking, I summarize what I heard.	"Let me see if I got everything you said. In summary, you said _____."	

RELATIONAL COMPETENCY	DESCRIPTION	ILLUSTRATION	RATING (1–10)
Expressing validation	When someone has finished speaking, I validate the logic of what they are saying, whether I agree with them or not.	"You make sense, and what makes sense is that when you experienced _____ [event], you would have thought/felt _____."	
Expressing empathy	When someone has finished speaking, I share with them the feelings I experienced them having or I imagine their feelings if they have not expressed them.	"Given all of that, I can see you that you feel _____ [if their feelings are physically visible]." "I can imagine you might be feeling _____ [some version of mad, sad, glad, or scared]."	
Mirroring, accuracy check, and expressing curiosity	If the speaker has other feelings, I mirror the additional feelings and check for accuracy and completion.	"And you also feel _____. Did I get that accurately? Are there other feelings?"	
Expressing gratitude	If I am the listener, I express gratitude to the speaker at the end of the conversation for sharing their thoughts and feelings with me.	"Thanks for sharing your thoughts and feelings with me."	
Expressing gratitude	If I am the speaker, I express gratitude to the listener at the end of the conversation for listening to my thoughts and feelings.	"Thanks for listening."	
TOTAL SCORE (MAXIMUM 240)			

Additional Resources

For relational educational opportunities by Harville and Helen, please visit www.HarvilleandHelen.com where you can:

- purchase books, e-books, and online courses;
- discover writings, podcasts, and invitations to special events, including live teleseminars with Harville and Helen;
- find updates on Harville and Helen's workshop and lecture schedule; and
- participate in a global mission of creating healthy relationships.

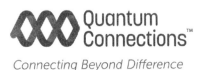

Quantum Connections brings the transformative power of Safe Conversations® Dialogue Methodology and Tools to small businesses, large corporations, global faith communities, educational institutions, and community organizations, along with individuals, couples, and families. Based in the neuro and quantum social sciences, Quantum Connections delivers comprehensive and highly structured training programs that are designed to foster the use of essential SC Dialogue skills in all interpersonal interactions—empowering people to talk to one another without criticism and listen without judgment to connect beyond difference. Our customers gain measurable value as high-performing teams eliminate silos and traditional company and cultural boundaries and move the organization from monologue to dialogue, which will, ultimately, result in significantly improved levels of employee engagement, retention, and inclusivity.

Developed and refined over four decades, the Safe Conversations Dialogue Methodology and Tools that form the foundation of Quantum Connections' training programs are the intellectual property of founders Harville Hendrix, PhD, and Helen LaKelly Hunt, PhD. Together, the proven methodology, time-tested tools, and skill-development practices used in Quantum Connections programs serve as the basis for the founders' bestselling book, *Getting the Love You Want*, with more than four million copies sold worldwide since 1988.

www.QuantumConnections.com

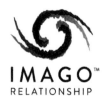

Imago Relationships International (IRI) was cofounded by Harville Hendrix, PhD, and Helen LaKelly Hunt, PhD, to help couples and individuals create strong and fulfilling relationships. More than twenty-five hundred Certified Imago Therapists are available in more than sixty countries. IRI is dedicated to providing the very best resources for therapists and laypersons seeking training to develop proficiency in the Imago relational method. The Imago Clinical and Facilitator Training provides an overview of the theory and essential skills for working with relationships.

www.ImagoRelationships.org

Notes

SESSION 7

1. William Congreve, *The Mourning Bride* (London: Bell's Edition, 1776), 7.
2. Sarah Keating, "The World's Most Accessible Stress Reliever," BBC, May 18, 2020, https://www
   .bbc.com/future/article/20200518-why-singing-can-make-you-feel-better-in-lockdown.
3. Daisy Fancourt, Lisa Aufegger, and Aaron Williamon, "Low-Stress and High-Stress Singing
   Have Contrasting Effects on Glucocorticoid Response," *Frontiers in Psychology* 6, no. 1242
   (September 2015): https://doi.org/10.3389/fpsyg.2015.01242.
4. Nick Stewart and Adam Lonsdale, "It's Better Together: The Psychological Benefits of Singing in
   a Choir," *Psychology of Music* 44, no. 6 (November 2016): 1240–1254, https://doi.org/10.1177
   /0305735615624976.
5. Gunter Kreutz et al., "Effects of Choir Singing or Listening on Secretory Immunoglobulin A,
   Cortisol, and Emotional State," *Journal of Behavioral Medicine* 27 (2004): 623–635, https://doi
   .org/10.1007/s10865-004-0006-9.
6. R. I. M. Dunbar et al., "Performance of Music Elevates Pain Threshold and Positive Affect:
   Implications for the Evolutionary Function of Music," *Evolutionary Psychology* 10 (2012):
   688–702, https://doi.org/10.1177/147470491201000403.
7. Rebecca Joy Stanborough, "10 Ways Singing Benefits Your Health," Healthline, November 10,
   2020, www.healthline.com/health/benefits-of-singing.
8. Fancourt, Aufegger, and Williamon, "Low-Stress and High-Stress Singing."

SESSION 8

1. Morella Hammer, interviewed by Sanam Hoon and Charlotte Legg, March 15, 2023.
2. Dawn Lipthrott, email to Sanam Hoon, January 29, 2024.
3. Helit Assa, interviewed by Sanam Hoon, April 14, 2023; Helit Assa, email to Sanam Hoon,
   February 1, 2024.
4. David Rudnick and Rabbi Elana Rosen-Brown, interviewed by Charlotte Legg, April 18, 2023.

About the
Authors

Harville Hendrix, PhD, began his career as a therapist and educator at the Pastoral Counseling Center of Greater Chicago in 1965, where he was clinical director. He received his doctorate in psychology and theology in 1970, and became a member of the faculty of Perkins Divinity School at Southern Methodist University in Dallas, Texas, where he taught for nine years. In 1979, he entered private practice as a therapist.

In 1977, Harville met Helen LaKelly Hunt and they married in 1982. They are cocreators of Imago Relationship Therapy, a couple's therapy, and coauthors of three *New York Times* bestsellers (*Getting the Love You Want, Keeping the Love You Find,* and *Giving the Love That Heals*); *Receiving Love, Making Marriage Simple, Doing Imago Relationship Therapy in the Space-Between*; and six other books on relationships. Imago Relationship Therapy has been featured on *The Oprah Winfrey Show* seventeen times, one of which won for her the "Most Socially Redemptive" Award for daytime talk shows. It has also been featured on many other major television shows and in countless radio shows, newspapers, and major magazines.

Harville and Helen founded the Institute for Imago Relationship Therapy to train therapists in the Imago process and to develop workshops for couples and singles. Later called the Imago International Training Institute, which has forty faculty members, the Institute has trained over twenty-five hundred therapists who practice Imago Relationship Therapy in over sixty countries, and nearly two hundred workshop presenters who conduct workshops around the world. These Imago professionals founded Imago Relationships Worldwide for professional growth and development and created an international Imago community.

In 2015, Harville and Helen cofounded Safe Conversations LLC, now Quantum Connections. This training institute teaches a relational intervention called Safe Conversations Dialogue, which is based on the latest relational sciences that can help anyone shift from conflict to connection. Harville and Helen believe that SC methodology and tools can contribute to a more relational world, with more gender and racial equity. To that end, the aim of Quantum Connections is to teach SC methodology and tools to 2.5 billion people (the tipping point of the world population in 2050) over the next thirty years, with the intention of facilitating that shift from our current "individualistic" civilization to a relational civilization, the fourth stage in human social evolution.

Harville is a graduate of Mercer University in Macon, Georgia, which awarded him an Honorary Doctorate of Human Letters. He holds a Master of Divinity from Union Theological Seminary in New York and a Master of Arts and a PhD in psychology and religion from the School of Divinity at the University of Chicago. Harville is the recipient of several honors, including the Outstanding Pastoral Counselor of the Year Award (1995) from the American Baptist Churches, the 1995 Distinguished Contribution Award from the American Association of Pastoral Counselors, and, jointly with Helen, the Distinguished Contributors Award from the Association for Imago Relationship Therapy. He is a Diplomate in the American Association of Pastoral Counselors and has been a clinical member of the American Group Psychotherapy Association and the International Transactional Analysis Association. He is a former board member of the Group Psychotherapy Foundation.

Harville and Helen have a blended family of six children and eight grandchildren. They live and work in Dallas, Texas, and New York City.

Helen LaKelly Hunt, PhD, earned her doctorate in women's history from Union Theological Seminary in New York City. She is a cocreator with her husband, Harville Hendrix, of Imago Relationship Theory & Therapy and cofounder of Imago International Training Institute, which has a teaching faculty of forty members, and of Imago Relationships Worldwide, which supports the growth and practice of Imago Relationship Therapy in over sixty countries by over twenty-five hundred therapists.

In 2015, Helen cofounded with Harville an organization called Safe Conversations LLC, now known as Quantum Connections. This training institute teaches SC methodology and tools, a relational intervention based on the latest relational sciences that can help anyone shift from conflict to connection. Helen believes that SC can contribute to a more relational world, with more gender and racial equity.

In addition to her partnerships with Harville in the cocreation and distribution of Imago Relationship Therapy and Safe Conversations, Helen is one of a small army of women who helped seed and develop the global women's movement. She cofounded the Texas Women's Foundation, the New York Women's Foundation, Women's Funding Network, and Women Moving Millions. For her achievements, she was inducted into the National Women's Hall of Fame in 1994 to the global women's movement and into the Smithsonian Institute for creating Women Moving Millions and her leadership in creative women's philanthropy.

Helen is sole author of *Faith and Feminism: A Holy Alliance*. Her latest book, *And the Spirit Moved Them: The Lost Radical History of America's First Feminists*, shares the inspiring story of the abolitionist feminists. Given her great interest in psychology, she has coauthored several books with Harville on Imago Therapy. These include three *New York Times* best-sellers (*Getting the Love You Want, Keeping the Love You Find*, and *Giving the Love That Heals*); *Receiving Love, Making Marriage Simple, Doing Imago Relationship Therapy in the Space-Between*; and six other books.